Vectors and Vector-Borne Zoonotic Diseases

Edited by Sara Savić

Published in London, United Kingdom

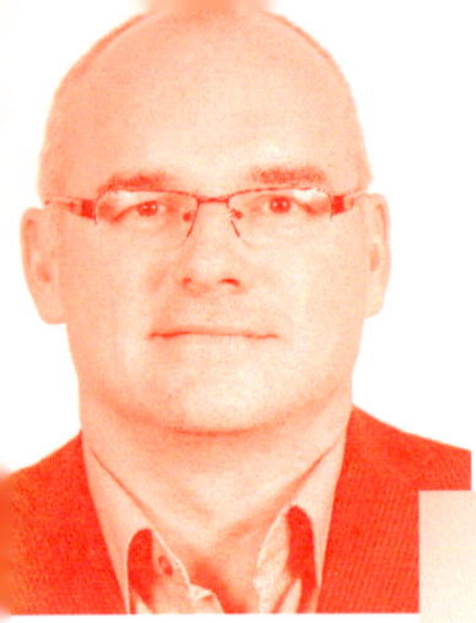
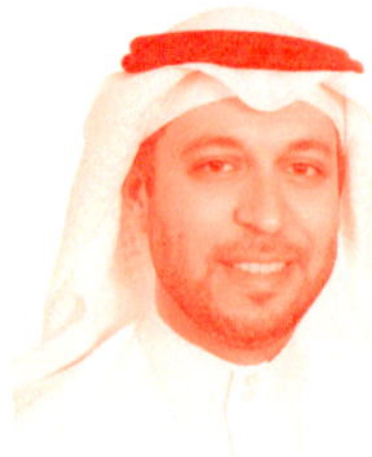
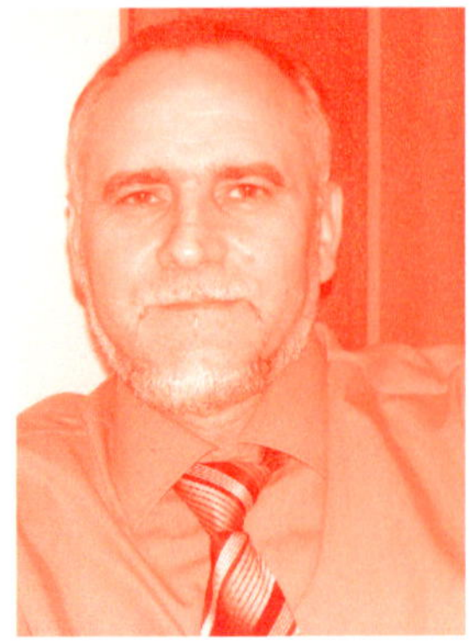
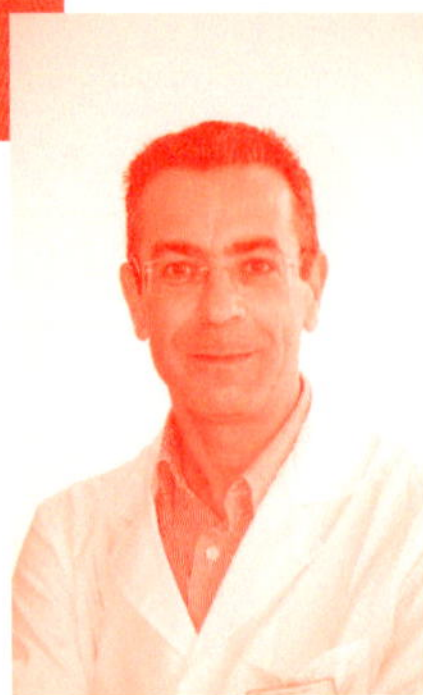
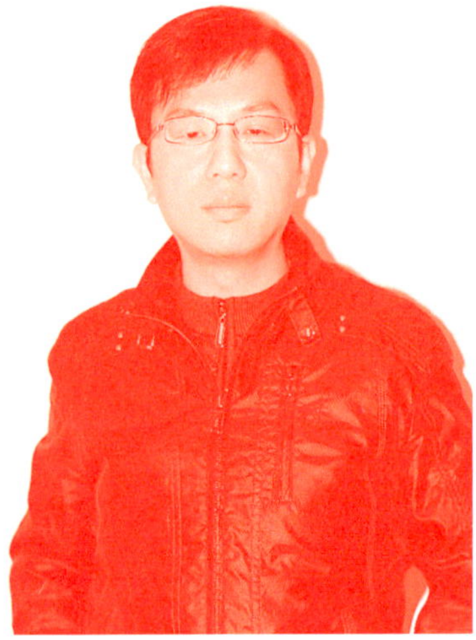
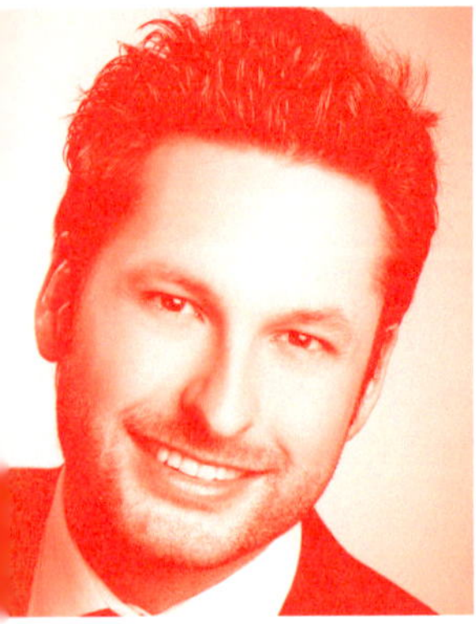
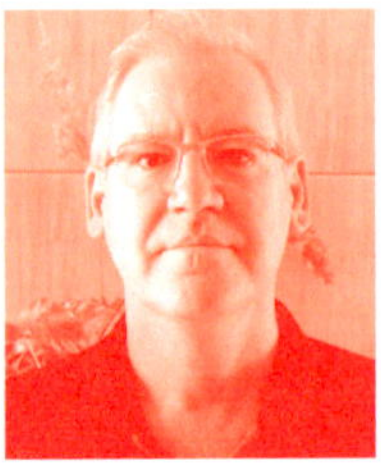

IntechOpen

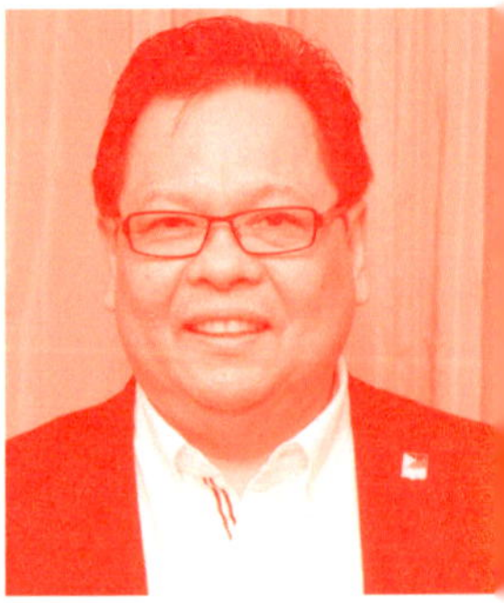
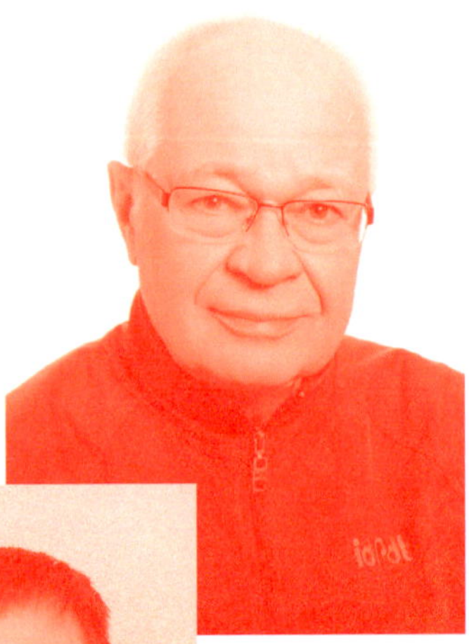
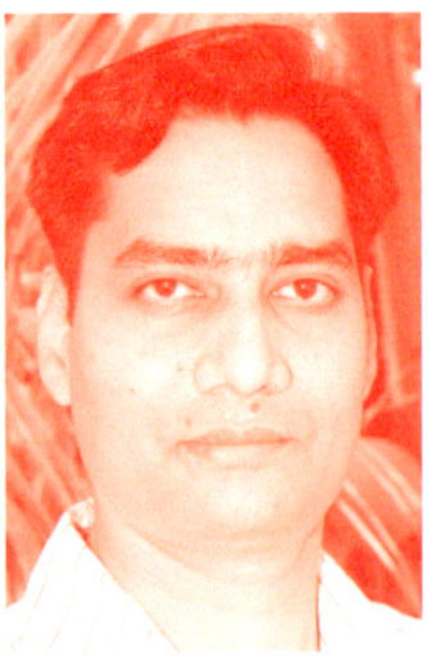
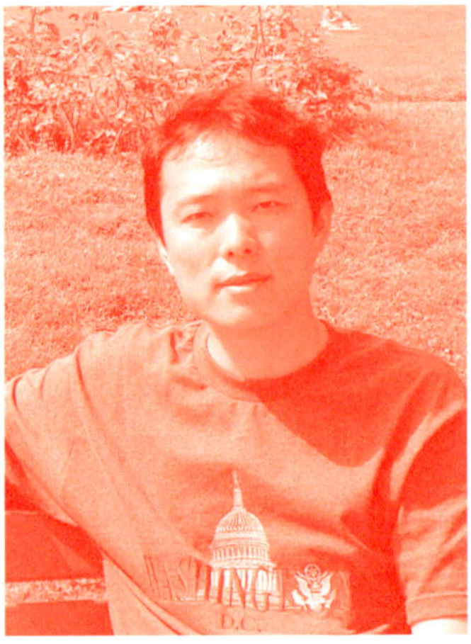
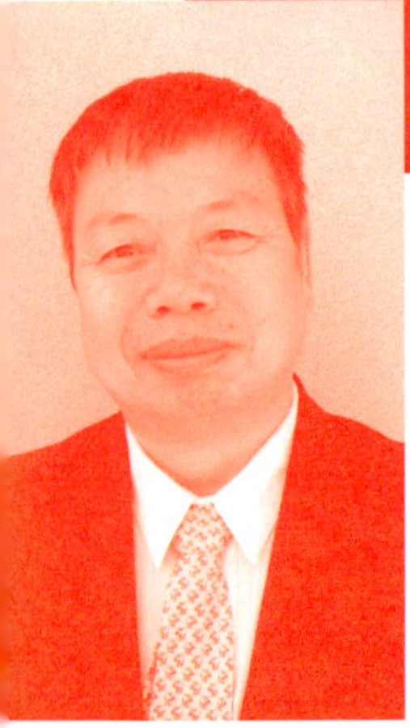
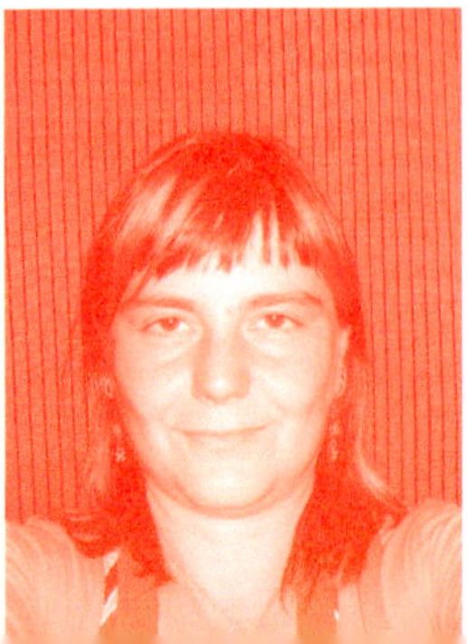

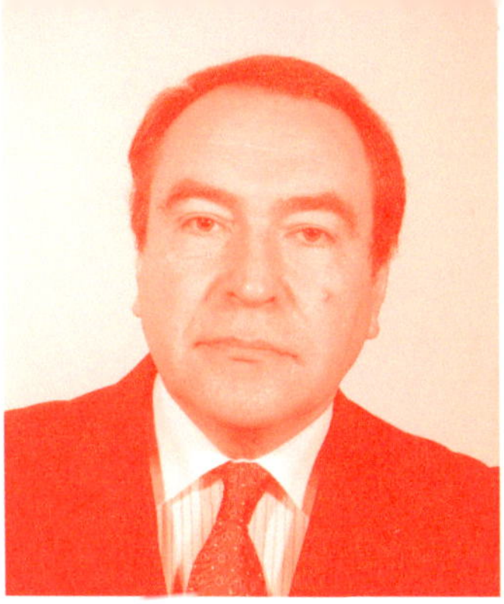
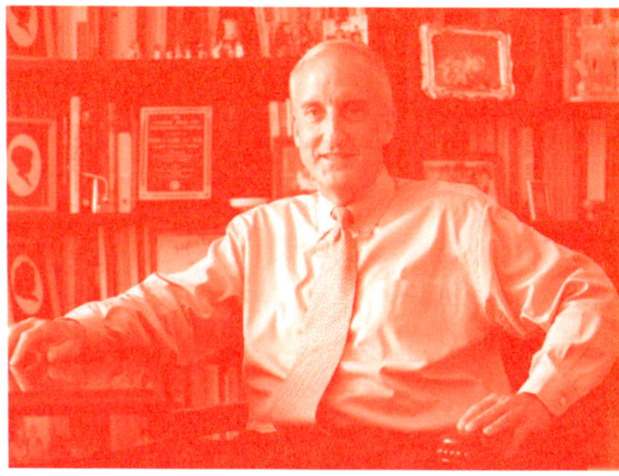
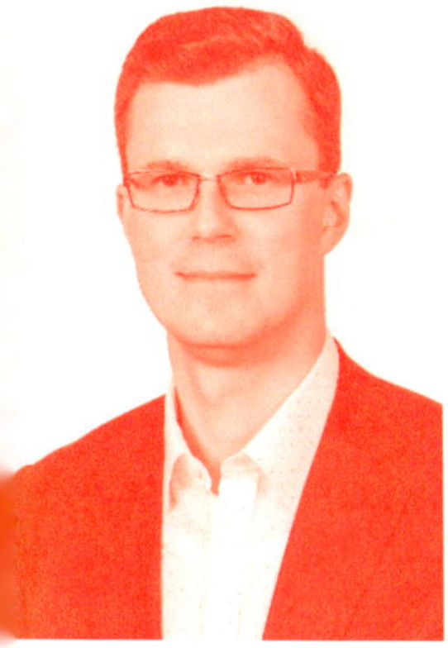
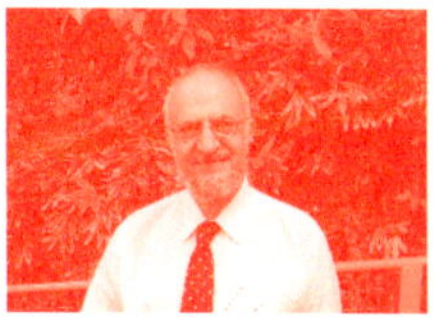
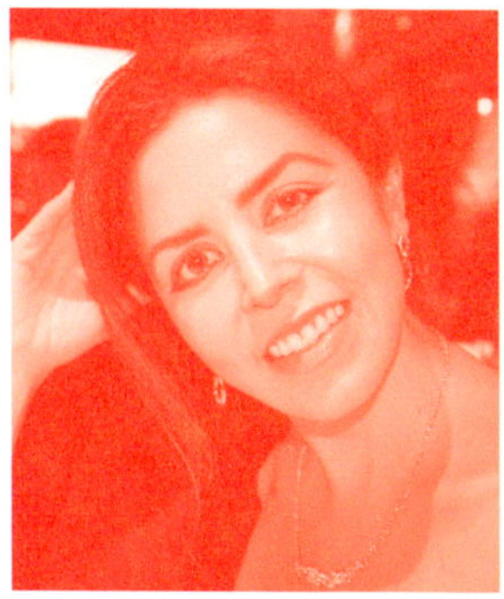

Supporting open minds since 2005

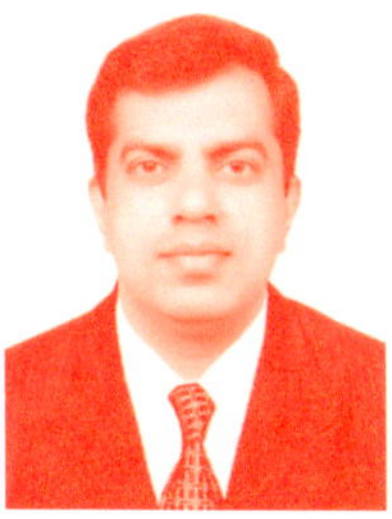
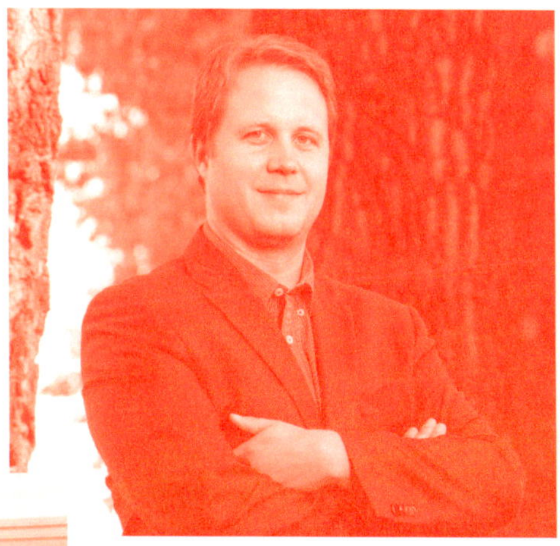
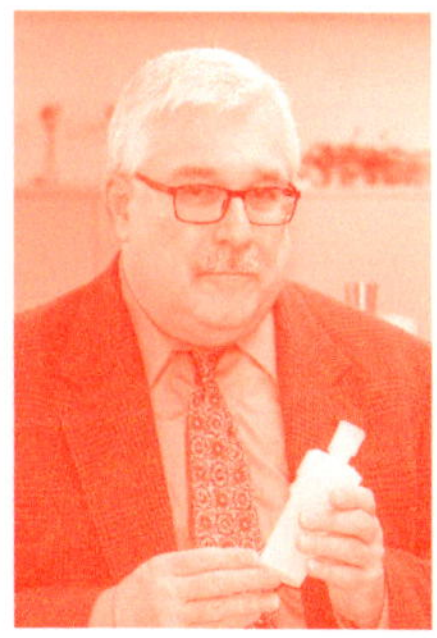
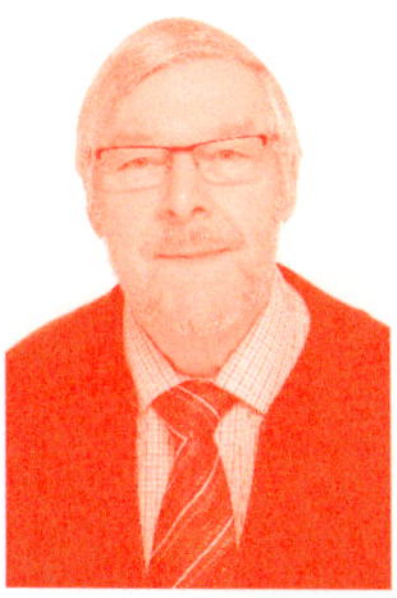
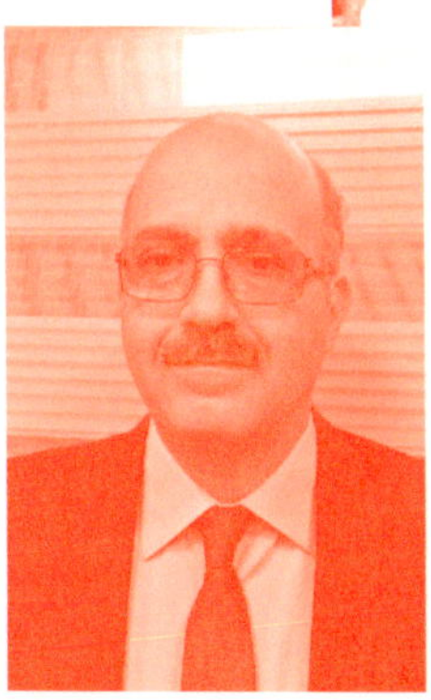
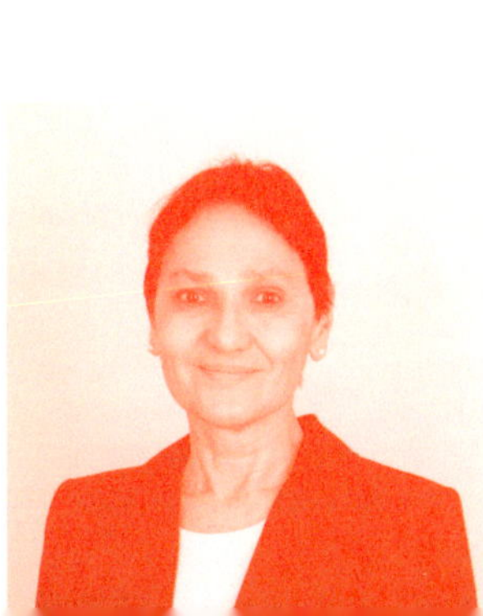
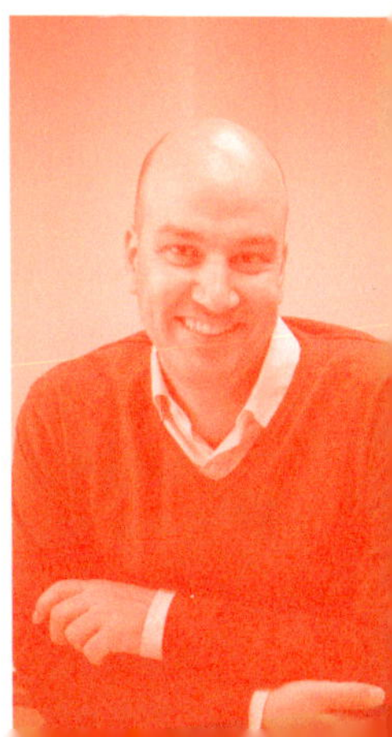

Vectors and Vector-Borne Zoonotic Diseases
http://dx.doi.org/10.5772/intechopen.77985
Edited by Sara Savić

Contributors
Iva Christova, Roberto Badaro, Daniel Motta, Frank Kirchner, Alex Santos, Nazli Ayhan, Remi N. Charrel, Biswadeep Das, Sayam Ghosal, Swabhiman Mohanty, Ana Sofia Santos, Maria Margarida Santos-Silva, Mümtaz Güran, Sara Savic

First published in London, United Kingdom, 2019 by IntechOpen
IntechOpen is the global imprint of INTECHOPEN LIMITED, registered in England and Wales, registration number: 11086078, The Shard, 25th floor, 32 London Bridge Street
London, SE19SG - United Kingdom
Printed in Croatia

British Library Cataloguing-in-Publication Data
A catalogue record for this book is available from the British Library

Additional hard copies can be obtained from orders@intechopen.com

Vectors and Vector-Borne Zoonotic Diseases
Edited by Sara Savić
p. cm.
Print ISBN 978-1-78985-293-6
Online ISBN 978-1-78985-294-3

For EU product safety concerns:
IN TECH d.o.o., Prolaz Marije Krucifikse Kozulić 3, 51000 Rijeka, Croatia, info@intechopen.com or visit our website at intechopen.com.

Meet the editor

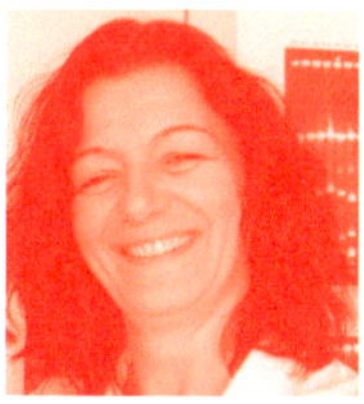

Sara Savić, PhD, DVM, is a researcher working in a diagnostic laboratory within the Scientific Veterinary Institute "Novi Sad" in Novi Sad, Serbia. Her main work is based on the diagnostic procedures for zoonotic diseases and vector-borne zoonoses. Dr. Savić completed her PhD degree on Diagnostics of Lyme disease in dogs and ticks, and then turned her interests and career towards other vector-borne diseases important for public health and One Health issues. The significance of multidisciplinary and transdisciplinary work has become most interesting during the past decade. Her expertise is in bacterial and parasitic vector-borne zoonoses, especially in blood parasites. Dr. Savić has published over 100 publications so far as a leading author or as a coauthor in different scientific journals or at conferences.

Contents

Preface

This book is about a group of diseases that can infect humans and animals and that are transmitted by vectors, and are called vector-borne zoonotic diseases. These diseases and the vectors that carry the causative agents are known terms in human and animal medicine, because of their effect on public health in general. In this book, the authors have tried to show which vectors and diseases are the most interesting, having in mind that their spreading represents a danger to public health.

Vectors and Vector-Borne Zoonotic Diseases is not meant just for veterinarians, but for medical doctors and entomologists too. It is intended to be used by experts and also by students, animal owners, nature lovers, etc. The book has several sections: "Introduction," "Vectors," "Vector-Borne Diseases and Pathogens," and "Vector Control." Each of the sections is about one stage of vector-borne diseases. Each group of authors has dedicated their work to one of the topics with key roles on pathogens or vectors that are of great public health interest in their country or region.

The "Introduction" is about the terms that are used in the book and the current state of knowledge on vector-borne diseases: why are they spreading and which factors can influence their appearance. The section on "Vectors" has two chapters: one is about mosquitoes that probably carry the largest number of different pathogens and the other is about a specific tick as a vector. In the section on "Vector-Borne Diseases and Pathogens" the authors share their experiences with certain vector-borne diseases that represent a public health threat in their countries. The authors deal with the actual dangers associated with vector-borne pathogens, which are increasing all the time. The section on "Vector Control" is just the tip of the iceberg...it is possible to devote a whole book just to this topic.

This book is the work of scientists and researchers as a contribution to the general knowledge and sophisticated expertise of vectors and vector-borne zoonotic diseases. With this book, we hope to broaden reader's knowledge, point out the existence of some vector-borne diseases, and show an interest in any new achievements in this area of research, with the aim to upgrade the knowledge of general public health from a One Health perspective.

As the editor, I would like to dedicate this book to all the researchers, experts, colleagues, students, and others working hard protecting the public health status.

Sara Savić, PhD, DVM
Senior Research Associate,
Scientific Veterinary Institute "Novi Sad",
Department for Serology, Immunology, and Biochemistry,
Novi Sad, Serbia

Section 1

Introduction

Chapter 1

Introductory Chapter: Vectors and Vector-Borne Pathogens around Us

Sara Savić

1. Introduction

The book "Vectors and Vector-Borne Zoonotic Diseases" is about the vectors of diseases and the pathogens they can carry and transmit. The topic of vector-borne diseases is of high interest among many researchers around the world. There are more and more pathogens discovered or they are discovered in locations where they were not found before. There are also more and more hosts where the pathogens are discovered in, and there are several reasons for that.

2. The factors of the discovery of new and old vector-borne diseases

In our modern times, it is possible to travel across the world in a day. Today one can reach a destination in less than 36 or even 24 h, for which in the past several days or a week was needed. Also, people travel more because of the globalization of business or different vacation options and very often they take their pets with them—again, across the globe.

Besides that, today there are many highly developed diagnostic laboratory methods which are:

- sensitive and can detect a very small part of the pathogens (DNA);
- specific for a certain pathogen; and
- available to most of the laboratories in the world.

These methods are based on molecular diagnostic procedures and have a possibility to detect new pathogens in different kind of samples and to detect different strains of the same pathogen.

There is also a factor of global warming and the adjustment of vectors to the climate changes. Some vectors in order to complete their life cycle need a certain temperature of the environment. Over a decade ago, some vectors could be found only in the Mediterranean region and now they can be found all the way in the Balkans. There was also seasonality in the appearance of some vectors, like ticks were not to be found from November until March in the countries with continental climate. Nowadays, in some countries, ticks can be found all around the year and they can also be found in north European countries. It seems like the vectors have a fantastic ability to adjust to climate changes, new locations, new hosts, and new pathogens, which all together makes them perfect organisms for spreading the disease.

3. The terms vector and vector-borne disease

The subject of the book Vectors and Vector-Borne Pathogens is not only both vectors and pathogens that can be found in them but also the diseases that they can cause in animals or humans.

Vector is an invertebrate animal (most usually an arthropod) that transmits infectious agents to vertebrates. In infectious disease epidemiology, vector is an insect or any living carrier that transports an infectious agent from an infected individual, or its wastes to a susceptible individual or its food or immediate surroundings [1]. In short, it is an organism that transmits a pathogen from one host to another.

Vector-borne disease can be transmitted differently:

1. Mechanical way of pathogen transmission—includes just mechanical transmission of the pathogen by a crawling or flying insects, on their legs, feet or wings, or proboscis, or by passage of the pathogens through their gastrointestinal tract. There is no multiplication or development of the pathogen within the mechanical vector, so no port of the pathogens life cycle occurs in the mechanical vector.

2. Biological way of pathogen transmission—involves part of the pathogens life cycle to occur within the vector: propagation (multiplication), stage development, or some combination of them is needed to occur in the vector, before it can transmit the infective form of the pathogen to the host (an animal or human). The incubation period is therefore needed after the infection so that this process can occur, before the vector becomes infectious and is able to transmit the infection. The pathogen within the vector can also be transmitted vertically to the next generation of the vector (transovarian transmission). Also, a trans-stadial transmission can occur, meaning that the pathogen can be transmitted from one stage of the life cycle to another, like for example, from the nymph to the adult. When the pathogen is "ready" within the vector, the transmission of the pathogen from vector to host can be done in different ways. The pathogen can be injected from a salivary gland with the fluid during the blood meal of the vector. Or, it can be transmitted by the regurgitation process, or deposition on the skin of feces or other material that can penetrate through a bite wound or an area of traumatized skin from scratching or rubbing [1]. Transmission like this usually occurs by an infected non-vertebrate host and it is not a simple mechanical carriage by a vector. Whichever role the arthropod takes, it is labeled as a vector.

In order to transmit the disease, a vector has to be competent for it. Vector competence is the ability of a vector to acquire, maintain, and transmit microbial agents. Not all blood-sucking arthropods are vectors (transmitters) of disease agents [1].

One same vector-borne disease can be seen as a neglected or endemic one, or an emerging or a reemerging one. It all depends on the geographic appearance of the disease (country or a region) and the relation of the countries public health toward that disease.

Neglected diseases are the ones that there is at least an evidence of the pathogen present in the environment, but there is no official acknowledgment of the threat from the disease. On the other hand, once the pathogen is in the environment, with appropriate vectors, hosts, and climatic conditions, the disease can develop to its full capacity causing clinical symptoms in animals and humans and then the disease becomes endemic for a certain region/country. Endemic diseases are maintained in a population without the need of external outputs. Emerging disease is either a newly recognized, clinically distinct disease or a known infectious disease whose reported incidence is increasing in a given place or among a specific population. They are rapidly increasing in incidence or geographic range.

4. The origin, purpose, and significance of the book

This book is a product of scientific and research work of many authors. The data presented are mostly from the original work done by the authors. But, it is presented in the way to be available not only to the scientific audience, but also for education and information. It is a collection of different experiences, cases, and studies with a same general topic on vector-borne diseases. The purpose of the book is to show how much public health can be endangered by the pathogens in vectors which can cause a disease and how much are vector-borne diseases present in our everyday life. It can also be used for education of students in order to show which vector-borne diseases represent a major public health threat in different parts of the world.

The book "Vectors and Vector-Borne Zoonotic Diseases" should point the readers to comprehend the One Health approach or aspect when thinking about vectors and vector-borne diseases. One Health concept recognizes the optimal health of people as being connected to the health of animals and the environment. It unites the collaborative effort of multiple disciplines working locally, nationally, and globally to attain optimal health for people, animals, and our environment. One Health approach considers the role of changing environments with regard to infectious and chronic disease risks affecting humans and nonhuman animals. The book is indicating a One Health point of view to be adopted by the reader. All the experiences shown in the book are somehow related intentionally or non-intentionally to One Health approach in the work of authors. The authors in the book represent multidisciplinarity and transdisciplinarity in work with vector-borne diseases.

The nature of the book is transdisciplinary, but united around one topic—vector-borne diseases. It shows the research work of different groups of experts, like entomologists, virologists, medical doctors, veterinarians, epidemiologists, microbiologists, and others, and all of them working and serving in the protection of Public Health. They all contributed to the book with a purpose for the readers to acknowledge the existence of different vector-borne diseases in different parts of the world and how people cope with them worldwide.

This book should be considered as very important book of experience because of its practical use in situations when public health has been endangered by vector-borne diseases. It also shows the reality and significance of transdisciplinary and multidisciplinary research groups with the same interest and passion that they all share for vectors or vector-borne diseases. There is also the educational role of the book, with a purpose to teach the young researchers about vectors and vector borne zoonotic pathogens and their significance within the public health.

Author details

Sara Savić
Scientific Veterinary Institute "Novi Sad", Novi Sad, Serbia

*Address all correspondence to: sara@niv.ns.ac.rs

Reference

[1] EurNEgVEc One Health Dictionary—A Product of a COST Action TD1303 European Network for Neglected Vectors and Vector Borne Infections. Available from: https://www.eurnegvec.org/publications/other/EurNegVecDictionary.pdf

Section 2

Vectors

Chapter 2

Aedes: What Do We Know about Them and What Can They Transmit?

Biswadeep Das, Sayam Ghosal and Swabhiman Mohanty

Abstract

Mosquitoes thrive mostly in the tropics and act as the vectors of some of the most debilitating human diseases caused by bioagents. Among the plethora of mosquitoes, *Aedes* transmit arboviruses, which have caused large-scale outbreaks throughout the world. Stegomyia is the most important subgenus of *Aedes*, which includes *Ae. aegypti* and *Ae. albopictus* vectors that are widespread and transmit a wide variety of arbovirus belonging to Togaviridae with the genus Alphavirus (Sindbis virus, equine encephalitis viruses, chikungunya virus), Flaviviridae with the genus Flavivirus (yellow fever virus, dengue 1–4 viruses, West Nile virus, Japanese and St. Louis encephalitis/SLE-viruses) and the Bunyaviridae with the genera Bunyavirus (California Group), and Phlebovirus (Rift Valley fever). In India, dengue and chikungunya are the most important arboviral diseases transmitted by *Ae. aegypti* and *Ae. albopictus* in recent time. Chikungunya and dengue are acute debilitating arthritogenic and hemorrhagic (dengue) disease, caused by enveloped single-stranded RNA virus belonging to Alphavirus and Flavivirus, respectively. In this chapter, we will comprehensively delineate the taxonomy of *Aedes* mosquitoes, their geographical distribution, evolutionary biology of chikungunya and dengue viruses, mechanism of transmission, and proposed vector control strategies against *Aedes* mosquitoes.

Keywords: *Aedes*, taxonomy, vector borne disease, chikungunya, dengue, phylogeny, *Wolbachia*

1. Introduction

1.1 *Aedes* mosquito: overview

1.1.1 Brief account on mosquitoes

Mosquitoes are one of the most important groups of insects, because of their significance to humans and animals as vectors of some of the most debilitating diseases. They are small, two-winged insects and found mostly living in the humid tropics and subtropics. Mosquitoes are widely investigated by the researchers because they act as the vectors for a variety of pathogens and parasites including viruses, bacteria, protozoans and nematodes.

1.1.2 Mosquito systematics and classification of Aedes

Mosquitoes are placed in the family Culicidae, suborder Nematocera of the order Diptera (the two-winged flies or true flies). The Culicidae family contains over 3200 species and are divided into 3 subfamilies: Anophelinae, Culicinae, and Toxorhynchitinae [1]. Subfamily Toxorhynchitinae comprises a single genus, *Toxorhynchites* comprising about 76 species. *Toxorhynchites* are not considered as medically important, because both sexes of Toxorhynchitinae possess a proboscis which curves backwards, thereby making them incapable of piercing the skin and transmitting disease in comparison to Anophelinae and Culicinae. There are three genera Anophelinae subfamily, however; only *Anopheles* is of medical importance [2]. There about 60 species of *Anopheles* mosquitoes which are known to be vectors of malaria [3]. Culicinae are the major vectors of arboviruses and filariasis. Medically most important genera in subfamily Culicinae are *Culex*, *Aedes*, *Mansonia*, *Haemagogus,* and *Sabethes* [3, 4].

There are more than 2500 species of Culicinae, with Aedes being the major genus, belonging to tribe Aedini [4]. Aedini is the largest tribe of family Culicidae with currently comprising 1240 recognized species. The traditional classification of Aedini is based on the concept of identifying few genera and numerous subgenera [5, 6]. The tribe Aedini was considered as a natural group; however, it was noted that some members showed affinities with all other higher-level taxa of subfamily Culicinae [6]. Species of the tribe Aedini vary extremely and are difficult to identify at the genus level because of overlapping suites of similar morphological features. Hence, different combinations of attributes are required to clarify the majority of the genera, subgenera and species. General characteristics of the tribe include the presence of toothed ungues (tarsal claws) and a pointed abdomen in most females. The traditional classification of Aedini prior to the end of the twentieth century comprised nine genera and 50 subgenera [7, 8]. *Aedes* was by far the largest genus comprising about 1000 species and further subdivided into 41 subgenera. Reclassification of genus *Aedes* began with the elevation of *Verrallina* and *Ayurakitia* to generic status [9, 10], followed by subsequent separation of the remaining subgenera into genera *Aedes* and *Ochlerotatus* [11]. Huge controversies

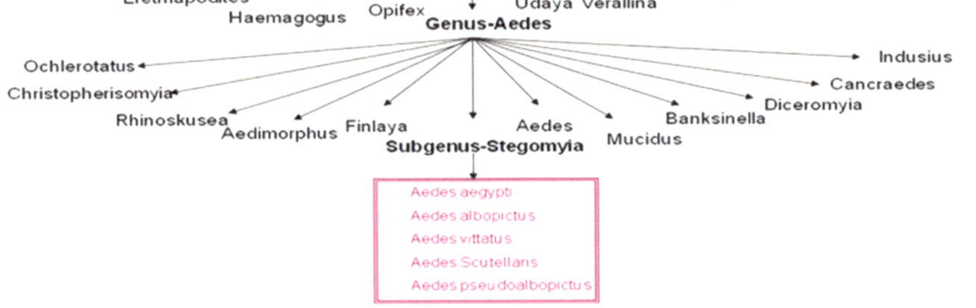

Figure 1.
Classification of Aedes up to the subgenus level showing few important species of the medically important subgenus Stegomyia.

have aroused after the reclassification, especially after upgrading *Ochlerotatus* group to generic status, due to which correct classification of *Aedes* still remains a paradigm [12]. Genus *Aedes* is further subdivided into several subgenera comprising over 900 species (**Figure 1**). Subgenus *Stegomyia* comprises most of the medically important *Aedes* species which are best known vectors of yellow fever, dengue fever, chikungunya fever and some forms of filariasis and other viral diseases [3].

1.1.3 The life cycle of Aedes mosquito

Like all other Dipterans, *Aedes* mosquitoes are holometabolous insects, meaning that they undergo a complete metamorphosis process, starting with an egg, larva, pupa, and adult stage.

The adult life span can range from 2 weeks to a month depending on environmental conditions [13]. Most species are unautogenous, that means after copulation the females have to take a blood meal to complete egg development: *Eggs*: after taking a complete blood meal, females produce on an average 100–200 eggs per batch; however, the number of eggs produced is dependent on the size of the blood meal. Eggs are laid on damp surfaces in areas likely to temporarily flood, such as tree holes and man-made containers, and are laid singly, rather than in a mass. Generally, eggs are positioned at varying distances above the water line, and the female mosquito does not lay the entire clutch at a single site; instead, it spreads out the eggs over two

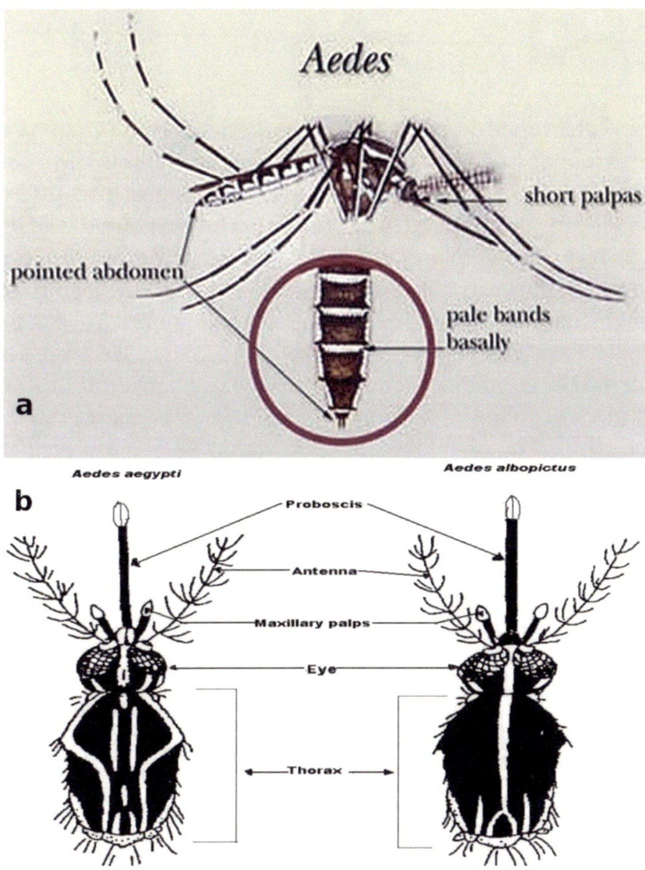

Figure 2.
(a) General morphological parts of an Aedes mosquito and (b) thorax of adult female Ae. aegypti and Ae. albopictus mosquito.

or more sites [14]; *Larvae*: mosquito larvae are often called "wrigglers" or "wigglers," because they appear to wiggle sporadically in the water upon disturbance. *Aedes* larvae breathe oxygen through a posteriorly located siphon that is held above the water surface, whereas the rest of the body hangs vertically. Larvae are generally found around homes in puddles, pots, cement tanks, tree holes, tires, or within any receptacle retaining water. Larval development is dependent on temperature. The larvae transition through four instars, spending a small duration in the first three instars, and up to 3 days in the fourth instar. Fourth instar larvae are approximately eight millimeters long and are vigorous feeders. Males generally pupate earlier because they develop faster than females. If the environmental temperatures are cool, *Ae. aegypti* can remain in the larval stage for months until the water supply is sufficient [14]; *Pupae*: after the fourth instar, *Aedes* larvae enter the pupal stage. Pupae, also called "tumblers," do not feed and take around 2–3 days to develop. Adults emerge by ingesting air to expand the abdomen thus splitting open the pupal case and emerge head first; *Adult*: *Aedes* adults can be remarkably distinguished from other mosquitoes by observing the whole body, which is striped, and so called "decorative mosquito" which is more distinct on the legs and scutellum, with short palpi and more or less pointed abdomen with pale bands. For example, adult *Ae. aegypti* and *Ae. albopictus* are often differentiated by the white scale bands on the dorsal part of the thorax. In case of *Ae. aegypti*, the pattern comprises two straight lines surrounded by curved lyre-shaped lines on the side. In contrast, a single broad line of white scales in the middle of the thorax is present in *Ae. albopictus* [15] (**Figure 2**).

1.1.4 Arbovirus and Aedes mosquitoes

Arboviruses (arthropod-borne-viruses) are defined as the viruses, which multiply within arthropods and can be transmitted by the arthropods to vertebrates. Usually, the arthropod gets infected by feeding on the blood from an infected vertebrate during viremia (virus circulation in the peripheral blood vessels), and then the virus can be transmitted to another vertebrate-host (horizontal transmission) after proliferation in the vector. Arboviruses can also be passed from one arthropod generation to another by transovarian transmission (vertical transmission). Several species of *Aedes* transmit arbovirus, which have caused large scale outbreaks throughout the world. *Stegomyia* is the most important subgenus of *Aedes* from medical point of view, followed by subgenus *Finlaya, Aedimorphus* and *Diceromyia*. *Ae. aegypti*, *Ae. albopictus*, *Ae. vittatus*, *Ae. scutellaris*, *Ae. pseudoscutellaris*, *Ae. polynesiensis*, *Ae. bromeliae* and *Ae. africanus* are the important vectors of subgenus *Stegomyia* that transmit several arboviral diseases across the world, out of which *Ae. aegypti* and *Ae. albopictus* are the most important vectors that are widespread and transmit a wide variety of arbovirus belonging mainly to three families: the Togaviridae comprising the genus *Alphavirus* (e.g., Sindbis virus, equine encephalitis viruses, chikungunya virus), Flaviviridae with the genus *Flavivirus* (e.g., yellow fever virus, dengue 1–4 viruses, West Nile virus, Japanese and St. Louis encephalitis/SLE-viruses) and the Bunyaviridae comprising the genera *Bunyavirus* (e.g., *California* Group), and *Phlebovirus* (Rift Valley fever) [16]. *Ae. poicilius*, *Ae. togoi*, *Ae. kochi*, *Ae. niveus*, and *Ae. harinasutai* of subgenus *Finlaya* are important vectors of arboviruses and microfilariae in the Oriental Region. *Ae. vexans* of the subgenus *Aedimorphus* has an extensive distribution in tropical Africa, Central America, Southeast Asia, and temperate regions of the Nearctic and Palaearctic Regions. Two species of the subgenus *Diceromyia*, *Ae. taylori* and *Ae. furcifer* have been implicated in the transmission of yellow fever virus and the spread of chikungunya virus in Africa [17].

In India, dengue and chikungunya are the most important arboviral diseases that are transmitted mainly by *Ae. aegypti* and *Ae. albopictus* and have caused massive and unprecedented outbreaks in recent times, thereby causing huge loss of lives and economic burden to the nation [18–20].

1.2 Chikungunya: overview

1.2.1 History and phylogenetics of CHIKV evolution

CHIKV was first isolated and characterized in 1953 during an epidemic of febrile polyarthritis in Tanzania (formerly Tanganyika) [21]. The word "chikungunya" comes from ChiMakonde, the language spoken by the Makonde people, an ethnic group in southeast and northern Mozambique meaning "that which contorts or bends up" and refers to the stooping posture of infected patients due to severe joint pain.

Since the 1953 Tanzania outbreak, CHIKV has caused outbreaks in various parts of Africa. The re-emergence of CHIKV epidemic in Africa was documented in 1999–2000 in Kinshasa where an estimated 50,000 persons were infected. The first documented Asian outbreak took place in 1958 in Bangkok, Thailand. Since then, many outbreaks have been recorded from Cambodia, Vietnam, Laos, Myanmar, Malaysia and Indonesia. There is historical evidence that chikungunya virus originated in Africa and subsequently spread to Asia [22]. Phylogenetic analysis of CHIKV virus sequences originally identified three distinct clades separated primarily by geography designated the West African, Central/East African (ECSA) and Asian genotypes. The Asian genotypes have a high degree of sequence identity among themselves whereas the African strains exhibit wider sequence diversity and have been shown to undergo genetic microevolutions even during the course of an epidemic [23]. Recent phylogenetic studies showed that the Indian Ocean and Indian subcontinent outbreaks were caused by virus strains of the Indian Ocean lineage (IOL), which evolved from the ECSA genotype [19, 24]. This lineage first emerged in Kenya in 2004, and subsequently spread to several Indian Ocean islands, India and Southeast Asia. The IOL strains involved in the Indian Ocean and Indian outbreaks possessed the initial adaptive mutation, E1-A226V [25], which is a major genetic determinant of adaptation of CHIKV to *Ae. albopictus* vector species and provides a plausible explanation for how this mutant CHIKV caused epidemics in regions lacking the more typical urban vector, *Ae. aegypti* [26]. Introduction of new viral strains, viz. IOL strains inevitably leads to the question whether particular genotypes of CHIKV are associated with higher virulence or severe disease. In addition, the lack of a suitable animal model for CHIKV makes it difficult to verify such hypotheses [27]. On the other hand, association of the re-emergence of endemic strains with the outbreaks leads to a different question that can be clarified only by a combination of classic epidemiology and comparative genomics: whether the viruses re-emerged due to environmental, population immunity and/or vectorial factors, or whether outbreaks were triggered by adaptive evolution of the virus that endowed it with an increase in fitness and virulence? Therefore, knowledge of the complete genetic blueprint of CHIKV is essential for clarifying these crucial questions.

1.2.2 Chikungunya virus (CHIKV): genome structure and organization

Chikungunya is an acute debilitating arthritogenic disease, caused by chikungunya virus (CHIKV) belonging to *Alphavirus* genus; family Togaviridae, which consists of *Alphavirus* and *Rubivirus* genera. Approximately, 40 *alphaviruses* can infect vertebrates such as humans, rodents, birds, and horses, along with invertebrates. Mosquito vectors are responsible for the transmission between species, thereby rendering *alphaviruses* to be considered as arboviruses. CHIKV is an enveloped particle and has a single-stranded RNA genome of positive polarity. The genome is approximately 11.8 kb in length [28]. Under electron microscopy in green monkey kidney (Vero) cells CHIKV particles reveal a characteristic *Alphavirus* morphology.

CHIKV genome consists of polyadenylated RNA and is capped, which encodes two open reading frames (ORFs). Two-third of the genome includes the 5′ ORF that encodes four nonstructural proteins, which are involved in genome replication, capping of RNA, polyprotein cleavage, etc., essential for viral replication. This region is expressed as an nsP1-3 or nsP1-4 polyprotein via cap-dependent translation, which is further cleaved by an nsP2-encoded protease. In context to the structural protein ORF, it is embedded in a subgenomic mRNA, and is translated into proteins via a cap-dependent mechanism. This structural ORF polyprotein is finally cleaved into capsid, envelope glycoproteins E1, and glycoprotein E2. The mature virion comprises 240 heterodimers of E2/E1, which are arranged as trimeric spikes on its surface, and has a diameter of 70 nm (**Figure 3**). After being translocated by the secretory pathway, these heterodimer spikes penetrate into the plasma membrane of infected cells, and cytoplasmic nucleocapsids containing the genomic RNA and 240 copies of the capsid protein bud from the cell surface for assembly of the virion envelope and envelope protein spikes [28].

During early infection, the nonstructural proteins are synthesized directly from the two third of genomic RNA as a P1234 polypeptide that is further cleaved to form Nsp1, Nsp2, Nsp3, and Nsp4 nonstructural proteins. Nsp1 protein is involved in the synthesis of minus-strand RNA, in addition to building association of the replication complex with cellular membranes. Nsp2 protein acts as a helicase and proteinase that cleaves the nonstructural polyprotein to form the individual

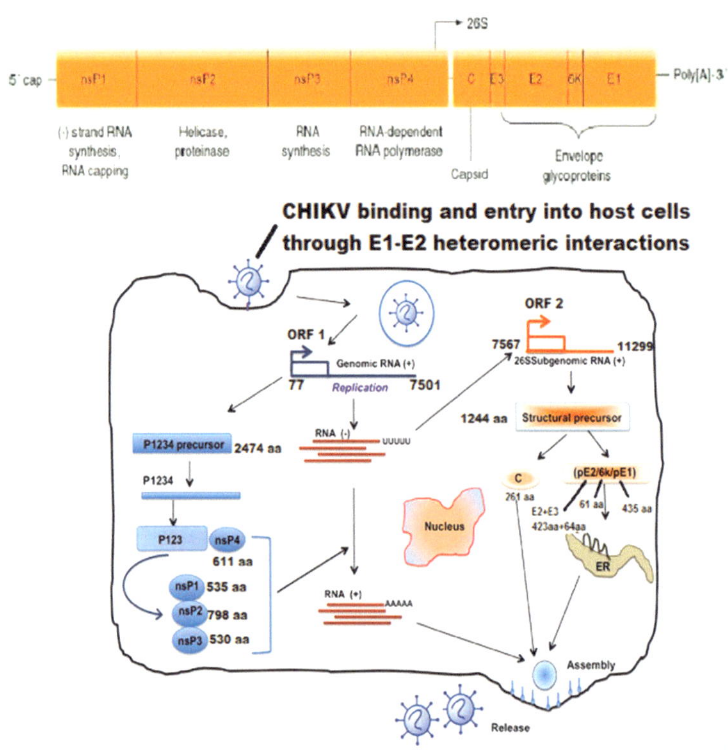

Figure 3.
CHIKV genome, binding, and entry into host cells followed by replication.

nonstructural proteins [30]. The function of Nsp3 in viral replication is largely unknown, however, it is probably involved in RNA synthesis [28]. Nsp4 interacts with the N terminal region and other nonstructural proteins and host factors, and acts as the viral RNA polymerase. The sub-genomic mRNA (26S) synthesizes single polypeptide that comprises the structural proteins, such as capsid, E3, E2, 6K and E1. These proteins are then cleaved co-translationally and post translationally to form the functional structural proteins. These structural proteins have important functions during virus replication and particularly, in the interaction with the host. Such interaction with the host was first presented by the production of antibodies that played important roles in the recovery from infection [31].

The region between the nonstructural and structural domains is called the "junction region," which enhances the transcription of an intracellular subgenomic 26S RNA. There are two other untranslated regions, along with the junction region; one at the 5′-end, which is required for the synthesis of the plus-strand [25], and the other at the 3′ end between the stop codon of the E1 gene and the poly (A) tail. This region is mainly involved in translation of viral proteins rather than in replication of the genomic RNA [28, 32].

1.2.3 Replication cycle of CHIKV

The interaction between the envelope proteins of CHIKV and receptors of host cells is required to penetrate into vertebrate cells. The cellular receptors for CHIKV are still unknown; however, in other Alphavirus the laminin receptor, glycosaminoglycans and DC-SIGN (CD209) molecules are involved in viral uptake [33]. The virus is transported into the cell by endocytosis of clathrin-coated vesicles. The activation of E1 protein from the E1-E2 complex is initiated because of the pH reduction of the vesicle, thereby initiating fusion of viral and endosomal membranes, resulting in the release of the nucleocapsid into the cytoplasm. Replication of CHIKV occurs in the cytoplasm. The first event is P1234 precursor polyprotein translation and RNA replication. P1234 polyproteins are directly translated from the viral genome, followed by the initiation of RNA replication through the synthesis of a complete minus-strand RNA, which serves as the template for the synthesis of the viral genome and for the transcription of 26S subgenomic plus-strand RNA from the internal promoter of the junction region. As both processes are interlinked, Nsp4 associates with P123 and other host factors to regulate the synthesis of minus-strand RNA, after cleavage from the P1234 polyprotein. This switching from genome replication to transcription of sub-genomic 26S positive-strand RNA is also regulated by the nonstructural proteins that were cleaved from the P123 polyproteins [34]. The 26S subgenomic RNA that serves as the mRNA translates the structural protein precursor, and further undergoes co-translational cleavage to become mature (C-E3-E2-6 k-E1). Autocatalytic cleavage of the N-terminal region of structural polyprotein precursor generates the capsid protein, followed by encapsidation of the viral genomic RNA, thereby, resulting in the rapid assembly of nucleocapsid cores in the cytoplasm. In parallel, E2 and E1 are transferred to the plasma membrane after being cleaved from the envelope polyprotein precursor. Finally, the packaging of the virus is performed in the cytoplasm by the assembly of nucleocapsid cores along with glycoproteins, and the virus is released by budding through the cellular membrane to form an enveloped virion [34].

1.2.4 Clinical presentations of CHIKV

The most common symptom in chikungunya disease is painful polyarthralgia, mainly bilateral, symmetrical and culminates within few days usually affecting peripheral joints like ankles, toes, fingers, elbows, wrists and knees. The joints exhibit extreme tenderness and swelling with patients frequently reporting incapacitating pain that lasts for weeks or months. Other typical signs for CHIKV infection include fever, headache, retro-orbital pain, chills, weakness, lumbar back pain, joint stiffness, malaise, nausea and a rash that may or may not be accompanied by other signs and symptoms of the disease [35]. The acute illness lasts 3–5 days, with recovery in 5–7 days. The incubation period following the bite of an infected mosquito is short (2–6 days) and ends with a sudden onset of fever reaching as high as 104°F that may last up to 10 days. The fever almost always precedes the rash and joint pain and only very rarely has been reported as biphasic with recurrence noted on the fourth or fifth day of illness. The rash, appearing primarily on the trunk, face, and limbs of the body is visible on day 2–5 postinfection, and may last up to 10 days. Older patients with an history of rheumatism exhibit more severe symptoms in comparison to younger patients [36].

1.2.5 Pathogenesis and diagnosis of CHIKV

Detailed studies on the pathogenesis of the chikungunya fever are rare. It is hypothesized that after inoculation, primary viral multiplication occurs in lymphoid and myeloid cells. The arthropod vectors acquire the virus by sucking blood during this period. The virus, then spreads to the targeted organs and immune system starts functioning at this stage, leading to the activation of both humoral and cellular immunity. This response of the body leads to the development of clinical features of the disease [36].

The probable diagnosis of chikungunya fever can be made on the basis of the presence of the virus in the community, and a clinical trial of fever, rashes and arthralgia, which are suggestive of the illness. The virus produces neutralizing and haemagglutination inhibiting (HI) antibodies, which helps in serological diagnosis. HI test is the simplest diagnostic test; however, it identifies the group rather than specific virus. Confirmation of the illness is done by detection of the antigen or antibody to the analyte in the blood sample of patient [37]. Reverse transcriptase polymerase chain reaction (RT-PCR) is a confirmatory test for the identification of CHIKV. IgM capture ELISA is the most sensitive serological assay, and can distinguish the chikungunya from dengue. All virus isolation procedures need to be done under bio safety level 3 (BSL-3) precautions, although such precautions may not be necessary in the countries where CHIKV is endemic.

1.2.6 Transmission cycles of CHIKV

CHIKV is transmitted by mosquitoes belonging to genus *Aedes*. The mosquitoes considered to be the main vectors for CHIKV are *Ae. albopictus* and *Ae. aegypti* [3]. Continuous variations in the geographic distribution of these vectors have been documented in several studies. *Ae. aegypti* was considered to be the primary vector of CHIKV in most parts of the globe [38], whereas *Ae. albopictus* (common name Asian tiger mosquito) was considered to be the secondary vector and was restricted to Asia [38]. However, the recent reemergence of CHIKV in many parts of the world has been mainly associated with *Ae. albopictus* vector [19, 38]. Furthermore, reports indicate *Ae. albopictus* to replicate and transmit the old African genotype of CHIKV as well as the recent Indian Ocean strain of CHIKV better than those of *Ae. aegypti* and other *Aedes* species [39]. CHIKV is endemic in tropical regions of Africa and Asia, where the mechanisms of CHIKV transmission and maintenance appears to be very complex and vary significantly depending on the particular region where virus activity is detected.

1.2.7 CHIKV in African mosquito vectors

In Africa, CHIKV is believed to be maintained in a sylvatic as well as with urban/rural cycle involving wild nonhuman primates and forest-dwelling *Aedes* mosquitoes (**Figure 4**). Several field studies conducted in Senegal, Nigeria, Uganda, Tanzania, Cote d'Ivoire, Central African Republic and South Africa concluded that the main sylvatic vectors of CHIKV are probably *Ae. furcifer*, *Ae. taylori*, *Ae. africanus*, *Ae. luteocephalus* and *Ae. Neoafricanus* [32]. Based on the isolation frequencies, it appears that *Ae. furcifer* and *Ae. taylori* are more important in southern and western Africa, while *Ae. africanus* is the chief vector in central regions [35]. Laboratory studies have confirmed vector competence of *Aedine* sylvatic mosquitoes in Africa. In South Africa, the oral infectious dose of *Ae. furcifer* was 50% (OID_{50})—the titer of the virus in the blood meal sufficient to infect 50% of mosquitoes was found to be less than 6.2 log/ml resulting in a transmission rate of 25–32%. This is sufficient to sustain CHIKV transmission from velvet monkeys and baboons, which develop viremia up to 7–8 log/ml [41].

1.2.8 CHIKV circulation in Asian mosquito vectors

In contrast to Africa, only urban/rural CHIKV transmission cycle has been described in Asia (**Figure 4**). *Ae. aegypti* is the main vector of CHIKV and *Ae. albopictus* is believed to play a secondary role in several outbreaks. CHIKV epidemics in humans seem to be disconnected from zoonotic transmission, however; the recent study of seroprevalence to CHIKV infection among wild monkeys in the Philippines showed presence of anti-CHIKV IgG in 59.3% of animals tested, suggesting existence of a possible sylvatic transmission cycles [42]. Currently, it is believed that persistence of CHIKV in Asia results from viral migration back and forth among different locations sustained by the human-*Ae. aegypti* cycle [43].

The vectors responsible for viral transmission during these epidemics have not been definitely characterized. Both *Ae. aegypti* and *Ae. albopictus* are present in India and their epidemiologic significances for CHIKV transmission probably vary

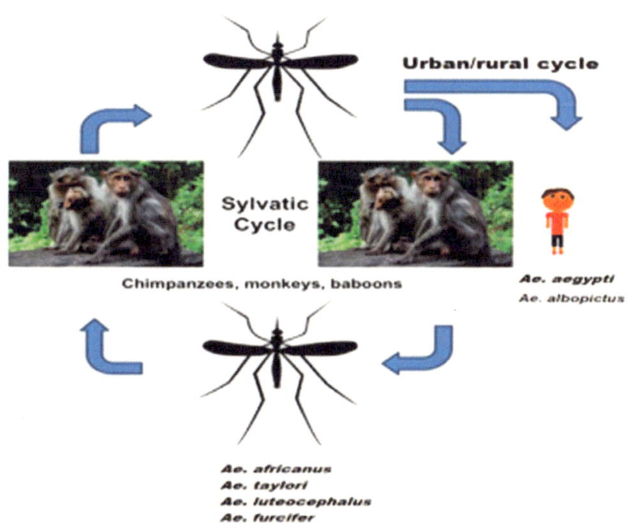

Figure 4.
CHIKV transmission cycle in Asia and Africa (modified from Thiboutot et al. [29, 40]).

dependent on the geographic location. Another intriguing feature of the 2006–2008 CHIKV epidemic in India, beside the magnitude, is the fact that this epidemic was caused by virus of the ECSA genotype. All previous outbreaks were caused by Asian genotype of CHIKV. It was proposed that this shift in viral genotype was the major factor in the re-emergence of Chikungunya in an unprecedented outbreak in India after a gap of 32 years [44].

1.3 Dengue: overview

1.3.1 History and geographic distribution of DENV

DENV is found in tropical and subtropical areas throughout the world, with prevalence in both urban and suburban areas. DENV is endemic in more than one-hundred countries with more than two-and-a-half billion people and around 40% of the world's population living in areas at risk for infection. The World Health Organization estimates that there are between fifty and one-hundred million DENV infections each year, causing hospitalization of five-hundred thousand people, and a death rate of two-and-a-half percent [45]. The earliest report of disease with dengue-like symptoms dates back to a Chinese encyclopedia of disease symptoms and remedies that was published from 265 to 420 A. D during the Chin Dynasty [46]. It is speculated that DENV was the etiological agent during disease outbreaks in the French West Indies in 1635, in Panama in 1699, and the Philadelphia epidemic of 1780 [47]. Reported cases of dengue disease were seen in 1779 and 1780 in Africa, Asia, and North America [48]. The first verified dengue epidemic occurred from 1953 to 1954 in the Philippines followed by a quick global spread of epidemics of DF/DHF. In the 1980s and 1990s, DENV continued to expand, and reached areas with mosquito vectors [49].

The very first report of the existence of dengue fever in India was in 1946 from US soldiers in Kolkata [50]. Since then, there was no significant dengue activity reported anywhere in the country for the next 18 years. In 1963–1964, an epidemic of dengue fever was reported from the Eastern Coast of India, further spreading northwards and reached Delhi in 1967 and Kanpur in 1968. Simultaneously, the DENV epidemic also engulfed the southern part of the country and gradually the whole country was affected by wide spread epidemics followed by endemic/hyperendemic prevalence of all the four serotypes of DENV. However, most dengue outbreaks in India were simple dengue fever with very rare cases of DHF/DSS epidemics. The first major wide spread epidemics of DHF/DSS occurred in 1996 in India, involving areas around Delhi and Lucknow, further spreading across the country [51, 52]. Since then, the epidemiology of DENV and its prevalent serotypes has been frequently changing in India.

1.3.2 Dengue virus (DENV)

Dengue virus (DENV) is a member of enveloped, positive-strand RNA viruses of the flaviviridae family. The flaviviridae family also includes West Nile virus, yellow fever virus, Japanese encephalitis virus, hepatitis C virus, and tick-borne encephalitis virus. Flaviviruses are transmitted to humans by arthropod vectors such as mosquitoes or ticks [49].

1.3.3 Dengue viral structure

There are four phylogenetically and genetically distinct, but antigenically related serotypes classified as DENV-1, DENV-2, DENV-3 and DENV-4. The dengue virion is a spherical particle, existing as either a 50 nm diameter immature particle or a mature 60 nm diameter particle with a lipopolysaccharide envelope. DENV genome is about 11 kb with a single ORF encoding three structural proteins: capsid (C), membrane (M), and envelope (E) and seven viral encoded nonstructural proteins: NS1, NS2A, NS2B, NS3, NS4A, NS4B and NS5 (Halstead, 2008). DENV RNA contains a type I cap structure (m7GpppAmpN2), located at its 5′-end, and lacks the poly (A) tail at its 3′ end. The DENV genome is surrounded with C proteins and forms the inner core. The structural proteins E and M are surface proteins on the virion envelope and the conformations of these proteins are used to distinguish between immature and mature virus. The immature virus is referred to as "spiky" as M proteins bound to a precursor membrane protein (pr) form heterodimers with E proteins that appear as "spikes" on the viral surfaces. In mature virions, the soluble pr is cleaved from M protein by furin, anchoring the M proteins and causing the pr protein to be absent in the mature viral membrane [53].

1.3.4 Dengue viral replication

DENV enters a variety of cells including macrophages, monocytes, and dendritic cells though cell endocytic vesicles. The first step in DENV infection is binding to the cellular receptors on the surface of the target cell like ubiquitous receptor (DC-SIGN). This interaction leads to the internalization of the virion via receptor-mediated endocytosis, resulting in the fusion of the virus with the endosomal membrane because of acidification, and finally releasing the viral genome into the cytoplasm. DENV genome is associated with rough ER (site of its translation), because the viral RNA can act as mRNA. Viral replication occurs in two steps: first, the positive-polarity RNA is copied to RNA of negative polarity that serves as a template for the synthesis of multiple strands of RNAs of positive polarity (amplification process); the positive-polarity RNA can then translate into proteins, for further RNA synthesis of negative polarity, or can become associated with structural proteins C, E, and M to form the viral progeny. Second, the immature virus particles travel to the Golgi apparatus in vesicles, where they undergo glycosylation, and are finally transported through secretory vesicles outside the cell (**Figure 5**). During the latter process, the furin cleaves prM in M to generate mature virions, which is the final step of viral morphogenesis [55]. The three main elements that are necessary for DENV replication are: *cis*-acting elements, trans-acting factors, and viral induced membranes.

1.3.4.1 Cis-acting elements

The *cis*-acting elements are mainly located at both ends of DENV genome in the 5′- and 3′-UTR. The cyclization sequences, as well as the upstream UAG region located at both ends of DENV genome and the downstream AUG region induce circularization of DENV genome. For an efficient negative-strand RNA synthesis, the secondary structure of the stem loop at the 3′-end (3′-SL), along with the secondary structure of SL structures within the 5′-UTR are essential. The initiation of viral replication occurs with the binding of NS5 (RNA dependent RNA-polymerase) to the 5′-UTR.

Trans-acting factors are of two types: viral *trans*-acting factors and cellular *trans*-acting factors.

Viral *trans*-acting factors: NS3 and NS5 (multifunctional and multidomain proteins, respectively) are the only proteins encoded by DENV possessing catalytic activities. NS5 has two main activities: RNA-dependent RNA-polymerase and methyltransferase. NS3 has protease, helicase, and nucleoside triphosphatase activities. NS3 functions by regulating its association with other viral proteins. NS1 and the small nonstructural proteins are required for anchoring the viral replication complex to the membranes of the endoplasmic reticulum.

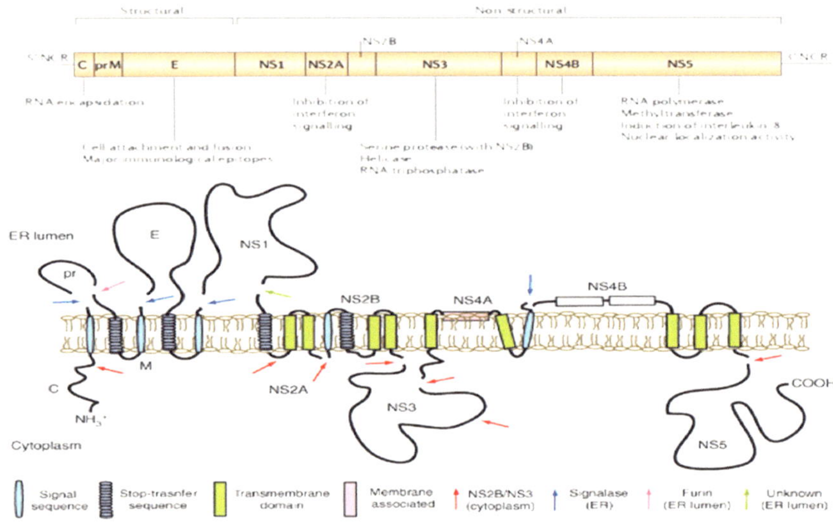

Figure 5.
Picture demonstrating: gene organization in DENV RNA genome (top), membrane topology and proteolytic cleavage sites of the transcribed polyprotein (bottom). Arrows denote the cellular and viral proteases, which process the immature polyprotein into ten separate proteins (modified from Perera and Kuhn [54]).

Cellular *trans*-acting factors: several cellular proteins, such as elongation factor 1a (EF1a), polypyrimidine tract binding protein (PTB), LA, calreticulin, PDI, and the heterogenous nuclear factors A1, A2/B1 and Q, have been found to bind to the 5′- or 3′-UTR of DENV. During DENV infection, PTB and La proteins translocate from the nucleus to the cytoplasm and act as the positive and negative regulators of viral replication, respectively. The YB-1 protein might participate in the switching from viral translation to replication or might have a role as an antiviral factor [54, 55].

1.3.4.2 Viral induced membranes (replication complex)

For the formation of the replication complex, proliferation and the generation of invaginations of the ER membranes are required initially, which are probably induced by NS4A and NS3 in conjunction with cellular and other viral proteins. Invaginations are mainly considered as the site for viral replication. The DENV RNA is exported to the convoluted membranes that might potentially store proteins and lipids required for DENV replication. Viral morphogenesis is initiated by the association of the RNA and the C protein generating nucleocapsids. The C protein accumulates around the lipid droplets in the ER. Accumulation of immature viral particles occurs in the lumen of dilated ER cisternae, which are then transported to the *cis*-Golgi for maturation (**Figure 6**) [56].

1.3.5. Classification and symptoms of dengue

Cases of symptomatic dengue have historically been classified by severity according to WHO guidelines first published in 1975, which differentiate between cases of dengue fever (DF), dengue hemorrhagic fever (DHF) and dengue shock syndrome [3] (**Figure 7**). However, dengue epidemiology has changed considerably since these guidelines were first published, leading to difficulties with the use of this classification system in a clinical setting. Examples of severe dengue that do not follow WHO criteria of DHF stratification are dengue with hemorrhage but without evidence of plasma leakage; dengue with shock syndrome without fulfilling all four DHF criteria; and severe dengue accompanied with organ dysfunction and a low level of plasma

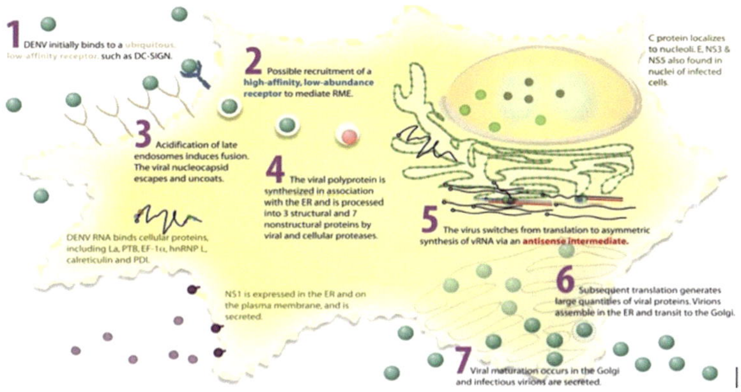

Figure 6.
Dengue replication cycle. Dengue enters a susceptible cell through receptor-mediated endocytosis. In endosomic vesicles, dengue virions are uncoated and release the genome into the ER. Viral RNA is translated into a polypeptide and processed to form viral proteins. Replication and viral assembly occurs in the ER, and the virions travel to the Golgi for modification and is exported via exocytic vesicles (adapted from Clyde et al. [56]).

leakage. In view of the above facts, recently the WHO Tropical Disease Research (TDR), 2009 [57] proposed a new classification of dengue, i.e., dengue (D), dengue with warning signs (DW) and severe dengue (SD) in order to re-evaluate the current classification for better management of high case fatalities. However, the previous

Dengue fever

Acute febrile illness with two or more of the following:
- headache
- retro-orbital pain
- myalgia
- arthralgia
- rash
- haemorrhagic manifestations
- leukopenia

and either supportive serology or proximity to laboratory confirmed cases.

Dengue haemorrhagic fever

The following indications must all be present:
- fever or a history of fever
- haemorrhagic tendencies evidenced by one or more of the following:
  - a positive tourniquet test
  - petechiae, ecchymoses or purpura
  - bleeding from the mucosa, gastrointestinal tract, injection sites or other locations
  - haematemesis or melaena
- thrombocytopenia (100,000 cells per mm3 or less)
- evidence of plasma leakage due to increased vascular permeability, manifested by at least one of the following:
  - a rise in the haematocrit equal to or greater than 20% above average for age, sex and population
  - a drop in the haematocrit following volume-replacement treatment equal to or greater than 20% of baseline
  - signs of plasma leakage such as pleural effusion, ascites and hypoproteinaemia

Dengue shock syndrome

All four of the above DHF criteria must be present, plus evidence of circulatory failure manifested by either of the following:
- rapid, weak pulse and narrow pulse pressure (<20mmHg)
- hypotension for age (systolic pressure <80mmHg for those less than 5 years of age, or <90mmHg for those greater than or equal to 5 years of age) and cold, clammy skin and restlessness

Figure 7.
Dengue case classification [3]. Dengue cases are classified as dengue fever (DF), dengue hemorrhagic fever (DHF), or dengue shock syndrome (DSS) according to the clinical observations shown in the figure.

classification of dengue [3] is still being followed in most countries for rapid diagnosis and prompt treatment of most cases with aggravated symptoms.

1.3.6 Pathogenesis and diagnosis of DENV

For the establishment of DENV infection in the patient, an incubation period generally occurs ranging between 3 and 14 days after a patient gets infected with DENV through the bite of an infected female *Aedes* mosquito. The patient subsequently experiences the painful febrile period when viremia is at its peak, which recedes in about 5–7 days after the onset of fever, coincident with defervescence. DHF/DSS usually develops during this time and the patient may develop intense clinical manifestations. If DHF develops, the patient may rapidly go into a state of shock and die within 12–24 hours if left untreated. After defervescence, laboratory diagnosis is based on IgG and IgM antibody detection. The disease progression for dengue is presented in the schematic form in **Figure 8**. The most commonly used diagnostic laboratory tests for DENV detection include those that detect DENVs, such as isolation by tissue culture and RT-PCR, and those that detect antibodies against the virus, such as enzyme-linked immunosorbent assay (ELISA), neutralization tests, haemagglutination inhibition (HI), and immunofluorescence (IF). Although the gold standard laboratory diagnosis of any flavivirus infection is isolation, and further characterization of the virus (for example by antigen detection) from the patient sample, it is a lengthy process and requires over a week for completion. In contrast, RT-PCR could be performed within hours and could therefore improve patient care. These detection methods are mainly used within approximately 10 days of the onset of symptoms because the virus is present in the sera typically till the duration of fever [3]. After this period, antibodies generated against DENV can be detected using serological methods. The antibodies neutralize DENV, and therefore, it is not possible to detect or culture the virus once the immune response is significantly underway.

1.3.7 Immune response and antibody-dependent enhancement (ADE)

Throughout his/her lifetime, a person can suffer from dengue infection four times (once for each of the four DENV serotypes). Both primary (first) and secondary (subsequent) infections by any DENV serotype can result in any of the two clinical manifestations: less severe DF or more severe DHF. A life-long immunity is conferred against the infecting serotype if primary infection occurs in a patient, along with a

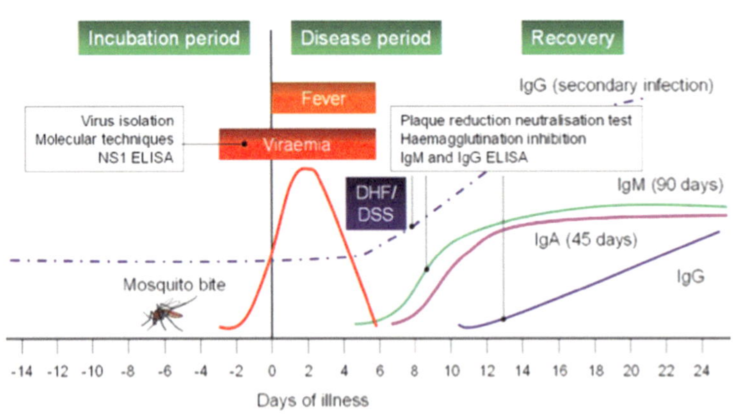

Figure 8.
Course of dengue infection and the timings and choices of diagnostic methods.

brief protection against infection by other DENV serotypes in the recovered patient. However, epidemiological data and some studies suggest that the immunity thus gained, after the lapse of the temporary cross-serotypic protection, increases the probability of an individual to develop DHF when infected by a second heterologous DENV serotype. A hypothesis that can explain this phenomenon is the antibody-dependent enhancement (ADE), which states that immunocomplexes are formed between the preexisting sub-neutralizing antibodies from the primary infection and the second infecting DENV serotype, which bind to the cells bearing Fcγ receptor (FcγR) (monocytes and B cells), thereby, leading to increased virus uptake and replication [58] (**Figure 9**).

1.3.8 Vectors and transmission cycles of DENV

Dengue is transmitted from person to person through the bites of infected female *Aedes* mosquitoes. DENV is believed to have been maintained in sylvatic/enzootic transmission cycles involving nonhuman primate hosts and vector species living in forests. The virus was first transmitted to humans when the two hosts (humans and nonhuman primate) came into contact, and was, thereafter established in continuous human-mosquito cycles in and/or around human population centers. Several species of the genus *Aedes* are known to transmit DENV; the principal vector is *Aedes aegypti*. The Australian naturalist, Thomas Lane Bancroft in 1906 first suggested that *Ae. aegypti* is the carrier of dengue fever based on epidemiological grounds [59]. *Ae. aegypti* is a day-biter that prefers to breed in domestic and peridomestic water containers. Its adaptation to human habitats and its desiccation-resistant eggs have allowed it to flourish in urban centers.

Ae. albopictus, commonly known as the Asian tiger mosquito is considered as the secondary vector of DENV. Koizumi et al., 1917 first identified its role as the dengue vector in semi-tropical regions in Taiwan [60]. *Ae. albopictus* serves as the primary vector for dengue in countries where *Ae. aegypti* is absent and as a maintenance vector in rural areas where both species coexist [61]. Moreover, ecology changes and global urbanization have caused major changes in the vectorial behavior of the two species, rendering *Ae. albopictus* to be the major vector of arboviral diseases like dengue and chikungunya in many countries, like India [19, 20]. In the Pacific islands, *Ae. polynesiensis* has been suggested as the primary dengue vector, whereas *Ae. scutellaris* was identified as the "jungle" vector for dengue [62]. In the continued absence of vaccines and specific treatment, effective vector control (either through fogging that kills adult mosquitoes, application of larvicides that target the aquatic stage of mosquitoes, source reduction that reduces their breeding habitat or biological control methods employing *Wolbachia* to hinder the fertility of mosquitoes) is currently the only practical method available for reducing the incidence of dengue disease [63].

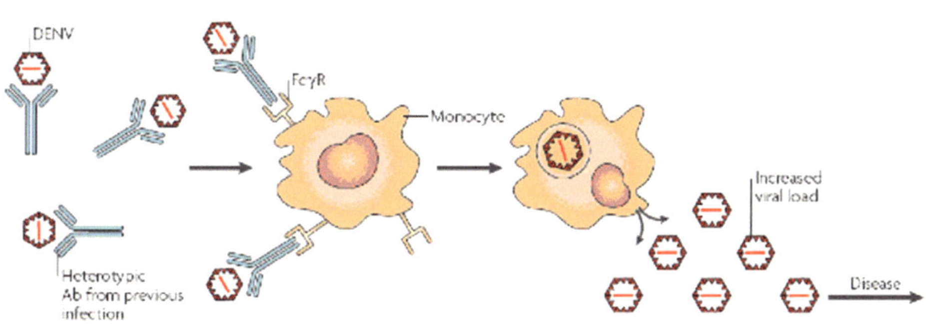

Figure 9.
Model for antibody-dependent enhancement (ADE) of dengue virus replication.

1.3.9 Role of phylogenetics in DENV evolution

DENV serotypes have been classified into multiple genotypes based on their genomic diversity. Genotype classification can often unveil the geographical origin of the dengue virus strains, except for the sylvatic genotypes. This has assisted in the temporal and spatial tracking of the virus transmission routes, which has served as the basis of molecular epidemiological studies, focusing on determining the causative agents of dengue epidemics, such as the introduction of new viruses and the result of re-emergence of endemic strains (**Figure 10**). Moreover, DENV has a tendency to evolve rapidly due to factors such as inter and intra serotypic recombination, mutation and ecological changes, thereby resulting in generation of new genotypes, which are more virulent, resistant and can cause massive outbreaks affecting large number of people. Introduction of such new viral genotypes inevitably leads to the question whether particular genotypes of DENV are associated with higher virulence or severe disease. To date, several diseases have often been associated with several DENV genotypes originating in Southeast Asia. The lack of a suitable animal model for the dengue disease poses challenges in confirming such hypothesis [64].

1.4 Vector control strategies

1.4.1 Conventional vector control

Vector control programs greatly depend on the use of chemicals such as insecticides like DDT, pyrethroids, organophosphates, and temephos. The annual demand of the insecticides amounts to more than 50,000 tons, with DDT being the most commonly used insecticide in the past. DDT, which is mainly used in indoor spraying for the control of vectors of malaria and visceral leishmaniasis, is forbidden in most of the countries today after the Stockholm Convention in 2001, when it was discovered to be dangerous to wildlife and the environment as it can remain in the environment and food chain for a considerably long time. Regarding other insecticides, most of them have undesirable effects besides their life-saving benefits. For example, vectors can become resistant and the nonbidegradability of the chemical frequently causes environmental damage. Although efforts have been conducted to develop a suitable vaccine against arboviral diseases like dengue and chikungunya,

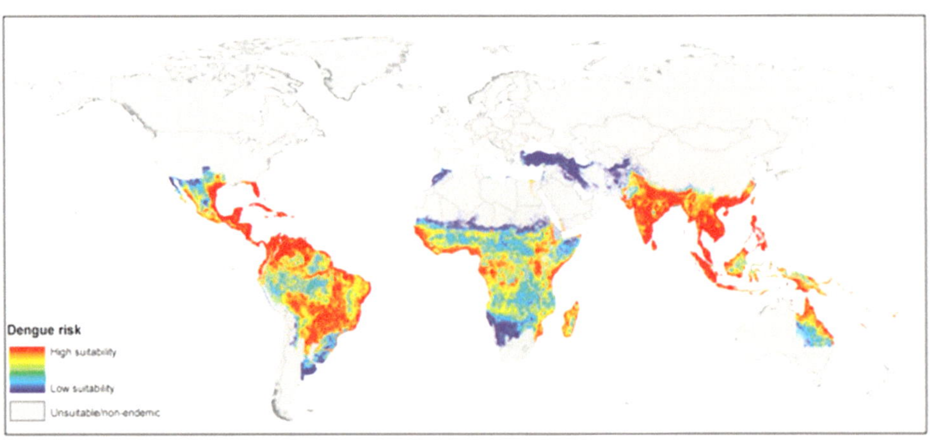

Figure 10.
Dengue risk map showing the highly suitable dengue epidemic areas around the world, depicting India to be a high-risk zone for dengue outbreaks (adapted from Simmons et al. [63]).

no vaccine has been developed with 100% efficacy to date. Therefore, the only means of reducing case fatality rate is early diagnosis and proper case management. The chief mode of controlling the disease is by eliminating the vector. It is of course much cheaper to prevent an outbreak of the disease than to diagnose and to treat the cases.

The major strategies for controlling *Aedes* vectors are: (1) reduction of *Aedes* breeding sites through environmental sanitation by the elimination of all nonessential water-containing receptacles. This is by far the most effective method in terms of long-term reduction of the mosquito population; (2) protection of water-containing receptacles by putting lids or covers to prevent egg laying by the mosquitoes; (3) release of larvivorous fish or other biological organisms as predators/parasites of larvae; (4) observation of a "Weekly Dry Day," i.e., the containers can be emptied at least once a week through generating awareness among the local population; (5) cleaning the containers before and after the rainy season can also contribute in reducing the mosquito populations and (6) space spraying, for example, with malathion against adult mosquitoes and larviciding with temephos.

1.4.2 Wolbachia: potential biocontrol agent

Wolbachia is a bacterium belonging to the tribe *Wolbachia* and family Rickettsiaceae and order Rickettsiales. They are a widespread group of bacteria commonly found in the reproductive tissues of arthropods. *Wolbachia* have attracted much attention by virtue of its ability to manipulate the reproduction of its arthropod hosts. Mosquito vectors such as *Aedes*, *Culex*, and *Anopheles* transmit a variety of diseases like dengue, filaria, Japanese encephalitis, and malaria. The vectors have gained resistance against insecticide and pesticides due to their variant mutation in genetic constitution. The continuous use of insecticides for control strategies increasingly faces the problems of high cost, increasing mosquito resistance and negative effects on nontarget organisms. *Wolbachia* have attracted scientific interest due to their ability to manipulate host reproduction, leading to distinct phenotypic effects in the host such as parthenogenesis, feminization, male killings and cytoplasmic incompatibility [65]. These modifications typically confer a reproductive advantage to infected individuals and allow the rapid spread of *Wolbachia* through a population [66, 67]. The most common effect of *Wolbachia* infection in mosquitoes is cytoplasmic incompatibility, which was first described in *Culex pipiens*, when infected male mosquitoes mated with uninfected female mosquitoes of the same species. The ability of *Wolbachia* to manipulate its host biology enables it to increase in frequency in host populations without the need for horizontal transmissions [68]. Hence *Wolbachia* can be used as a potential weapon against pests and the diseases they can carry.

Molecular phylogeny represents a great source of information for better understanding the evolutionary relationships among *Wolbachia* to analyze changes occurring in different organisms during evolution. The strain variation, of any *Wolbachia* species in mosquito populations is necessary for understanding the evolutionary mechanisms of *Wolbachia* genotypes in vector mosquitoes. Phylogenetic analysis of *Wolbachia* using different molecular markers is important to understand the evolution, pathogenesis and strain typing in areas having abundant arboviral vectors. Several molecular phylogenetic studies have been reported using *16S rRNA* gene, *ftsz* cell cycle gene, *wsp Wolbachia* surface protein gene, out of which *wsp* gene has been the most preferred for phylogenetic analysis [69].

Therefore, further studies of the natural occurrence and diversity of *Wolbachia* in the major *Aedes* vectors are of high interest. Ultimately, this will be useful for making strategies for vector control programmes by determining the specific strain of *Wolbachia* that is present in *Aedes* followed by artificial infection of *Wolbachia* into the major *Aedes* vectors that will effectively reduce their life span thereby reducing disease transmission.

Author details

Biswadeep Das*, Sayam Ghosal and Swabhiman Mohanty
KIIT School of Biotechnology, KIIT University, Bhubaneswar, India

*Address all correspondence to: biswadeep.das@kiitbiotech.ac.in

References

[1] Scott F. Biology. Glenview, Illinois: Scott, Foresman and Company; 1980. p. 689

[2] Service MW. Medical Entomology for Students. London: Chapman and Hall; 1996. p. 278

[3] WHO. World malaria situation in 1994. Part I. Population at risk. Weekly Epidemiological Record. 1997;**72**(36):269-274

[4] Kettle DS. Medical and Veterinary Entomology. New York: John Wiley and Sons; 1984. p. 658

[5] Edwards FW. *Genera Insectorum. Diptera, Fam. Culicidae*. Fascicle 194. Brussels: Desmet-Verteneuil; 1932

[6] Belkin JN. The Mosquitoes of the South Pacific (Diptera: Culicidae). Berkeley and Los Angeles: University of California Press; 1962

[7] Knight KL, Stone A. A Catalog of the Mosquitoes of the World (Diptera: Culicidae). 2nd ed. Vol. 6. Thomas Say Foundation. Entomological Society of America, Maryland, USA; 1977. pp. 1-611

[8] Ward RA. Second supplement to a catalog of the mosquitoes of the world: (Diptera: Culicidae). Journal: Mosquito Systematics. 1984;**16**: 227-270

[9] Reinert JF. Restoration of *Verrallina* to generic rank in tribe Aedini (Diptera: Culicidae) and descriptions of the genus and three included subgenera. Contributions of the American Entomological Institute (Gainesville). 1999;**31**:1-83

[10] Reinert JF. Restoration of *Ayurakitia* to generic rank in tribe Aedini and a revised definition of the genus. Journal of the American Mosquito Control Association. 2000;**16**:57-65

[11] Reinert JF. New classification for the composite genus *Aedes* (Diptera: Culicidae: Aedini), elevation of subgenus *Ochlerotatus* to generic rank, reclassification of the other subgenera, and notes on certain subgenera and species. Journal of the American Mosquito Control Association. 2000;**16**:175-188

[12] Harbach RE. The Culicidae (Diptera): A review of taxonomy, classification and phylogeny. Zootaxa. 2007;**1668**:591-638

[13] Maricopa County Environmental Services. Lifecycle and information on *Aedes aegypti* mosquitoes. Maricopa County, AZ. 2006. http://www.maricopa.gov/EnvSvc/VectorControl/Mosquitos/MosqInfo.aspx

[14] Foster WA, Walker ED. Mosquitoes (Culicidae). In: Mullen G, Durden L, editors. Medical and Veterinary Entomology. Sand Diego, CA: Academic press; 2002. pp. 203-262

[15] Barraud PJ. The Fauna of British India, Including Ceylon and Burma. Diptera, V, Family Culicidae, Tribe Megharini and Culicini. London: Taylor and Francis; 1934. pp. 217-246

[16] Murphy FA, Fauquet CM, Bishop DHL, Ghabrial SA, Jarvis AW, Martelli GP, et al. Virus Taxonomy–Classification and Nomenclature of Viruses. Sixth Report of the International Committee on Taxonomy of Viruses. Wien, New York: Springer-Verlag; 1995. p. 586

[17] Becker N, Petric D, Zgomba M, Boase C, Madon M, Dahl C, et al. Mosquito and their Control. 2nd ed. Heidelberg: Springer; 2003. p. 587

[18] Lahariya C, Pradhan SK. Emergence of chikungunya virus in Indian subcontinent after 32 years: A review. Journal of Vector Borne Diseases. 2006;**43**:151-160

[19] Das B, Sahu A, Das M, Patra A, Dwibedi B, Kar SK, et al. Molecular investigations of chikungunya virus during outbreaks in Orissa, eastern India in 2010. Infection, Genetics and Evolution. 2012;**12**:1094-1101

[20] Das B, Das M, Dwibedi B, Kar SK, Hazra RK. Molecular investigations of dengue virus during outbreaks in Orissa state, eastern India from 2010-2011. Infection, Genetics and Evolution. 2013;**16**:401-410

[21] Ross RW. The Newala epidemic. III. The virus: Isolation, pathogenic properties and relationship to the epidemic. The Journal of Hygiene. 1956;**54**(2):177-191

[22] Powers AM, Logue CH. Changing patterns of chikungunya virus: Re-emergence of a zoonotic arbovirus. The Journal of General Virology. 2007;**88**:2363-2377

[23] Volk SM, Chen R, Tsetsarki KA, Adams AP, Garcia TI, Sall AA, et al. Genome-scale phylogenetic analyses of chikungunya virus reveal independent emergences of recent epidemics and various evolutionary rates. Journal of Virology. 2010;**84**(13):6497-6504

[24] Tsetsarkin KA, Chen R, Leal G, Forrester N, Higgs S, Huang J, et al. Chikungunya virus emergence is constrained in Asia by lineage-specific adaptive landscapes. Proceedings of the National Academy of Sciences. 2011;**108**(19):7872-7877

[25] Tsetsarkin KA, Vanlandingham DL, McGee CE, Higgs S. A single mutation in chikungunya virus affects vector specificity and epidemic potential. PLoS Pathogens. 2007;**3**(12):e201

[26] Rougeron V, Sam IC, Caron M, Nkoghe D, Leroy E, Rogues P. Chikungunya, a paradigm of neglected tropical disease that emerged to be a new health global risk. Journal of Clinical Virology. 2015;**64**:144-152

[27] Leitmeyer KC, Vaughn DW, Watts DM, Salas R, Villalobos I, de Chacon, et al. Dengue virus structural differences that correlate with pathogenesis. Journal of Virology. 1999;**73**(6):4738-4747

[28] Strauss JH, Strauss EG. The alphaviruses: Gene expression, replication, and evolution. Microbiology and Molecular Biology Reviews. 1994;**58**(3):491-562

[29] Simizu B, Yamamoto K, Hashimoto K, Ogata T. Structural proteins of Chikungunya virus. Journal of Virology. 1984;**51**(1):254-258

[30] Vasiljeva L, Valmu L, Kaariainen L, Merits A. Site-specific protease activity of the carboxyl-terminal domain of Semliki Forest virus replicase protein nsP2. The Journal of Biological Chemistry. 2001;**276**(33):30786-30793

[31] Griffin DE, Johnson RT. Role of the immune response in recovery from Sindbis virus encephalitis in mice. Journal of Immunology. 1973;**118**(3):1070-1075

[32] Leathers V, Tanguay R, Kobayashi M, Gallie DR. A phylogenetically conserved sequence within viral 3′ untranslated RNA pseudoknots regulates translation. Molecular and Cellular Biology. 1993;**13**(9):5331-5347

[33] Ozden S. Human muscle satellite cells as targets of Chikungunya virus infection. PLoS One. 2007;**2**:e527

[34] Solignat M, Gay M, Higgs S, Briant L, Devaux C. Replication cycle of

chikungunya: A re-emerging arbovirus. Virology. 2009;**393**(2):183-197

[35] Jupp PG, McIntosh BM. Chikungunya disease. In: Monath TP, editor. The Arboviruses: Epidemiology and Ecology. Boca Raton (Florida): CRC Press; 1998. pp. 137-157

[36] McGill PE. Viral infections, α-viral arthropathy. Baillière's. Clinical Rheumatology. 1995;**9**:145-150

[37] Mourya DT, Thakare JP, Gokhale MD, Powers AM, Hundekar SL, Jaykumar PC, et al. Isolation of Chikungunya virus from *Aedes aegypti* mosquitoes collected in the town of Yawat, Pune district, Maharashtra state, India. Acta Virologica. 2001;**45**:305-309

[38] Enserink M. Infectious diseases. Massive outbreak draws fresh attention to little-known virus. Science. 2006;**311**(5764):1085

[39] Tsetsarkin KA, McGee CE, Volk SM, Vanlandingham DL, Weaver SC, Higgs S. Epistatic roles of E2 glycoprotein mutations in adaption of chikungunya virus to *Aedes albopictus* and *Ae. aegypti* mosquitoes. PLoS One. 2009;**4**:e6835

[40] Thiboutot MM, Kannan S, Kawalekar OU, Shedlock DJ, Khan AS, Sarangan G, et al. Chikungunya: A potentially emerging epidemic? PLoS Neglected Tropical Diseases. 2010;**4**:e623

[41] Paterson HE, McIntosh BM. Further studies on the Chikungunya outbreak in southern Rhodesia in 1962. II. Transmission experiments with the *Aedes Furcifer-Taylori* Group of Mosquitoes and with a member of the *Anopheles gambiae* complex. Annals of Tropical Medicine & Parasitology. 1964;**58**:52-55

[42] Inoue S, Morita K, Matias RR, Tuplano JV, Resuello RR, Candelario JR, et al. Distribution of three arbovirus antibodies among monkeys (*Macaca fascicularis*) in the Philippines. Journal of Medical Primatology. 2003;**32**(2):89-94

[43] Chevillon C, Briant L, Renaud F, Devaux C. The Chikungunya threat: An ecological and evolutionary perspective. Trends in Microbiology. 2008;**16**(2):80-88

[44] Dash PK, Parida MM, Santhosh SR, Verma SK, Tripathi NK, Ambuj S, et al. East central south African genotype as the causative agent in reemergence of Chikungunya outbreak in India. Vector Borne and Zoonotic Diseases. 2007;**7**(4):519-527

[45] World Health Organization. Dengue, Countries or Areas at Risk, 2011. WHO(South East Asia); 2012

[46] Nobuchi H. The Symptoms of a Dengue-like Illness Recorded in a Chinese Medical Encyclopedia. Kanpo Rinsho; 1979

[47] McSherry JA. Some medical aspects of the Darien schema: Was it dengue? Scottish Medical Journal. 1982;**27**:183-184

[48] Hirsch A. Dengue, a comparatively new disease: Its symptoms. In: Handbook of Geographical and Historical Pathology. London, United Kingdom: The New Sydenham Society; 1883. pp. 155-181

[49] Gubler DJ. Dengue and dengue hemorrhagic fever. Clinical Microbiology Reviews. 1998;**11**(3):480-496

[50] Karamchandani PV. Dengue group of fevers in India. Lancet. 1946;**1**(6386):92

[51] Afreen N, Deeba F, Naqvi I, Shareef M, Ahmed A, Broor S, et al. Molecular investigation of 2013 dengue fever outbreak from Delhi, India. PLOS Currents. 2014;**2**:6

[52] Tazeen A, Afreen N, Abdullah M, Deeba F, Haider SH, Kazim SN, et al.

Occurrence of co-infection with dengue viruses during 2014 in New Delhi, India. Epidemiology and Infection. 2017;**145**(1):67-77

[53] Heinz FX, Stiasny K, Allison SL. The entry machinery of flaviviruses. Archives of Virology. Supplementum. 2004;**18**:133-137

[54] Perera R, Kuhn RJ. Structural proteomics of dengue virus. Current Opinion in Microbiology. 2008;**1**(4):369-377

[55] Miller JL, deWet BJM, Martinez-Pomares L, Radcliffe CM, Dwek RA, Rudd PM, et al. The mannose receptor mediates dengue virus infection of macrophages. PLoS Pathogens. 2008;**4**(2):e17

[56] Clyde K, Kyle JL, Harris E. Recent advances in deciphering viral and host determinants of dengue virus replication and pathogenesis. Journal of Virology. 2006;**80**(23):11418-11431

[57] WHO/TDR. Dengue, Guidelines for Diagnosis, Treatment, Prevention and Control. Geneva: World Health Organization; 2009

[58] Whitehead SS, Blaney JE, Durbin AP, Murphy BR. Prospects for a dengue virus vaccine. Nature Reviews. Microbiology. 2007;**5**(7):518-528

[59] Cleleand JB, Bradley B, McDonald W. On the transmission of Australian dengue by the mosquito *Stegomyia fasciata*. The Medical Journal of Australia. 1916;**2**:179-184

[60] Kuno G. Research on dengue and dengue-like illness in East Asia and the Western Pacific during the first half of the 20th century. Reviews in Medical Virology. 2007;**17**(5):327-341

[61] Freier JE, Rosen L. Vertical transmission of dengue viruses by mosquitoes of the *Aedes scutellaris* group. The American Journal of Tropical Medicine and Hygiene. 1987;**37**(3):640-647

[62] Mackerras IM. Transmission of dengue fever by *Aedes (Stegomyia) scutellaris* walk in New Guinea. Transactions of the Royal Society of Tropical Medicine and Hygiene. 1946;**40**(3):295-312

[63] Simmons CP, Farrar JJ, Nqyun V, Wills B. Dengue. New England Journal of Medicine. 2012;**366**(15):1423-1432

[64] Rico-Hesse R. Dengue virus evolution and virulence models. Clinical Infectious Diseases. 2007;**44**(11):1462-1466

[65] Werren JH, Zhang W, Guo LR. Evolution and phylogeny of Wolbachia: Reproductive parasites of arthropods. Proceedings of the Biological Sciences. 1995;**261**(1360):55-63

[66] Joanne S, Vythilingam I, Yugavathy N, Leong C, Wong M, AbuBakar S. Unidirectional cytoplasmic incompatibility in Malaysian *Aedes albopictus* (Diptera: Culicidae). Annals of the Entomological Society of America. 2016;**109**(3):366-370

[67] Joanne S, Vythilingam I, Teoh BT, Leong CS, Tan KK, Wong ML, et al. Vector competence of Malaysian *Aedes albopictus* with and without Wolbachia to four dengue virus serotypes. Tropical Medicine & International Health. 2017;**22**(9):1154-1165

[68] Oliveira S, Villela DAM, Dias FBS, Moreira LA, Freitas RM. How does competition among wild type mosquitoes influence the performance of *Aedes aegypti* and dissemination of *Wolbachia pipientis*? PLoS Neglected Tropical Diseases. 2017;**11**(10):e0005947

[69] Sivan A, Shriram AN, Bhattacharya D, Vijayachari P. Prevalence of Wolbachia endosymbiont among field collected *Aedes albopictus* (Skuse) and phylogeny in south Andaman, Andaman and Nicobar Islands, India. Journal of Mosquito Research. 2015;**5**(22):1-10

Chapter 3

Ixodes ventalloi Gil Collado, 1936: A Vector Role to be Explored

Ana Sofia Santos and Maria Margarida Santos-Silva

Abstract

Ixodes Latreille, 1795 is the largest and broadest distributed genus of the family Ixodidae Murray, 1877. Its members are present in all zoogeographic regions, remote islands, and territories close to the poles. Plus, 63 species out of the 244 described have been recorded to feed on humans. Some are mega vectors, as those belonging to *Ixodes ricinus-I. persulcatus* complex, but others are so poorly studied that their vector role is difficult to access. This is the case of *Ixodes ventalloi* Gil Collado, 1936. This species is recorded in Northern Africa and Western Europe, mostly in Mediterranean basin countries, occurring along with other moisture-demanding ticks, as *Haemaphysalis* spp., *I. frontalis*, and *I. ricinus*. In fact, *I. ventalloi* not only shares vertebrate hosts (including humans) with the latter but may as well play a role in the enzootic cycle of some *Ixodes*-borne agents. This chapter updates information regarding this poorly studied tick, revising the available systematic, ecological, and microbiological data, discussing the potential public health relevance.

Keywords: *Ixodes ventalloi*, taxonomy, distribution, vertebrate hosts, tick-borne agents

1. Introduction

Ticks are a highly specialized group of obligate, bloodsucking, nonpermanent ectoparasitic arthropods of terrestrial vertebrates with a worldwide distribution. They present a hematophagic behavior in all active phases and parasitize mammals, birds, reptiles, amphibians, and occasionally man. Unique among Acari, ticks have a large body size being considered large mites with specialized mouthparts (hypostome) and specialized sensory structures on legs (tarsus I, Haller's organ) [1, 2]. These arthropods are among the most important vectors of human and animal disease. They are associated to the transmission of a great variety of pathogenic agents, including viruses, bacteria, and protozoa [3]. These pathogens are usually acquired by immatures, larvae, or nymphs, when ticks feed on infected hosts being maintained through their life and transmitted to naïve animals during the next blood meals, as nymphs and adults (horizontal transmission). Depending on the pathogen, ticks can also pass infection to the offspring (vertical transmission) or even to other ticks by feeding close to them (co-feeding). Ticks may also injure hosts without the involvement of infectious agents, just by the effects of salivary secretions, causing from a simple irritation to allergic reactions, toxicosis, and paralysis [4].

IntechOpen

Among the family Ixodidae Murray 1877, the genus *Ixodes* Latreille 1795 is the largest, the broadest distributed, and one of the most important *taxon* regarding tick-borne diseases. It comprises a total number of 244 species of which 63 have been recorded to feed on humans [5]. Its members are present in all zoogeographic regions, remote islands, and territories close to the poles. In Europe and North Africa, the genus *Ixodes* is represented by 25 species [5]. Within this genus, several ticks may be considered mega vectors as those that belong to the *Ixodes ricinus-I. persulcatus* complex, but others are so poorly studied that their vector role is difficult to access. This is the case of *Ixodes ventalloi* Gil Collado, 1936. This is a species that is infrequently targeted in field trials and laboratory collections are scarce. In Portugal, an expansion of its distribution was observed, most likely as a collateral result of concerted efforts to increase knowledge on the subject [6–12]. The recent interest of other specialists has also generated updated descriptions of the morphological features relevant for diagnosis and the first molecular characterization of *I. ventalloi* populations with the analysis of its phylogenetic position in the group *Ixodes* [13, 14]. Regardless of this, information on the vector role of *I. ventalloi* remains challenging to access and poorly understood. This chapter intends to update information on *I. ventalloi* in order to call attention to this insufficiently studied tick, revising the available systematic, ecological, and microbiological data, discussing the potential public health relevance.

2. One species three names: a question of synonymy

I. ventalloi was first described by Gil Collado based on the morphological characters of a female tick parasitizing an *Athene noctua* captured in Barcellona [15]. The identification of this small-sized *Ixodes*, among other features, was based on the presence of particularly large and curved auriculae (**Figure 1**), differentiating it from the other European species, as the author wrote "Las aurículas de la base del capítulo, muy típicas y de forma de "asta de touro" (...) la distinguen netamente de las espécies europeas (...)" [15]. In the following years of its description, *I. ventalloi* was misclassified and as a consequence, confusion arose regarding the morphological features and the ecology of this tick. *I. ventalloi* was either incorrectly ascribed as a new species, *I. thompsoni*, or confounded with *I. festai* and used for the redescription of the latter species mistaking both entities, as detailed by Gilot and Perez [16]. *I. festai*, originally described by Rondelli in 1926 based on the analysis of a female specimen found parasitizing a Libyan *Alectoris barbara*, is a bird-associated tick contrasting with the more permissive nature of *I. ventalloi*, as revised bellow in this chapter. Several works mention *I. thompsoni* and *I. festai sensu* Arthur as a synonym of *I. ventalloi*, but the definitive validation of this species was only achieved with the studies of Gilot, Morel and Perez [16–18].

Detailed descriptions of relevant morphological features have been subsequently updated, in some cases supported by illustrations and microscope images to better assist acarologists in *I. ventalloi* identification [14, 19–21]. Moreover, the application of mitochondrial DNA analysis using molecular targets, such as 12S rRNA, 16S rRNA, cytochrome *c* oxidase subunit 1 (*cox1*), has proven useful to complement the traditional morphological identification [12–14]. It also enabled the study of the population genetic structure. The molecular characterization of 92 *I. ventalloi* adults collected in cats from Lipari Island (Southern Italy) revealed the presence of a great genetic variability with the identification of eight haplotypes for 16S rRNA and 16 haplotypes for *cox1*, clustering in two sister clades—genogroup A, comprising 71% of the samples and genogroup B [13]. Interestingly, 16S rRNA sequences

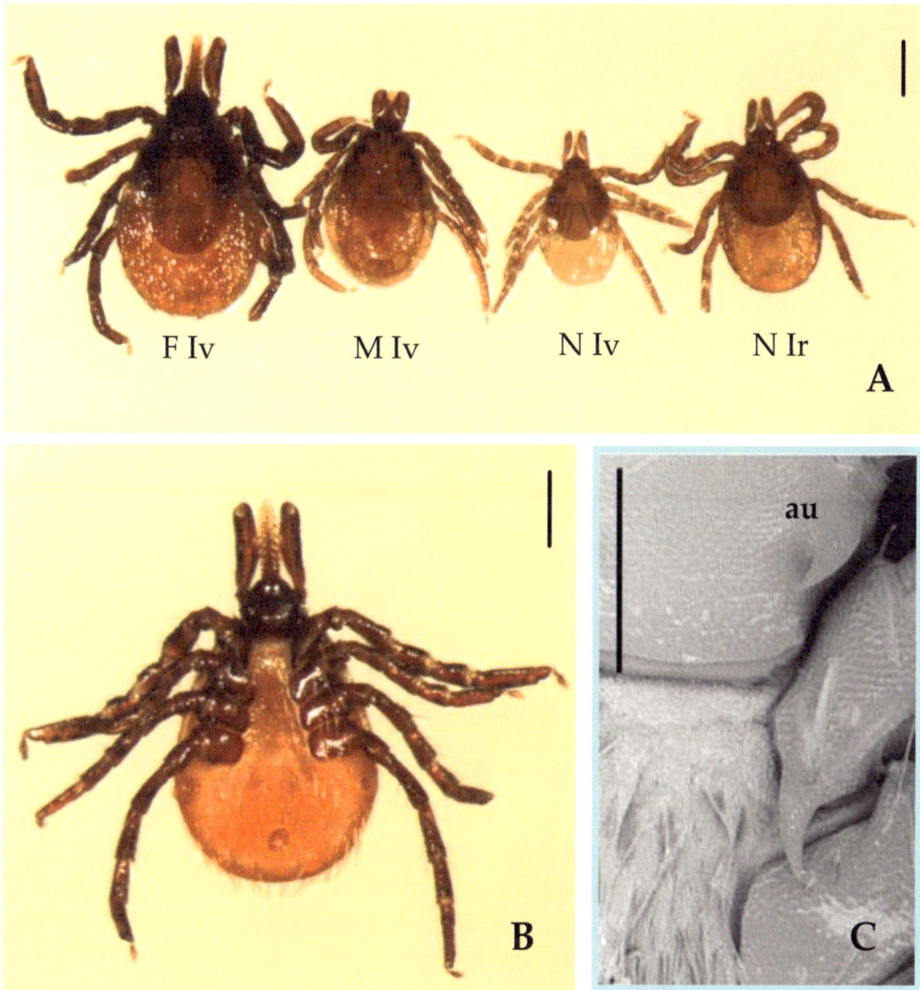

Figure 1.
Morphological features of Ixodes ventalloi: (A) Size comparison of questing I. ventalloi female (F Iv), male (M Iv), and nymph (N Iv) with a questing Ixodes ricinus nymph (N Ir), dorsal view, scale bar 2 mm; (B) ventral view of a questing I. ventalloi female, scale bar 2 mm; (C) scanning electron microscopy detail of the recurved auriculae (au), the hallmark feature first pointed by Gill Collado [15] for differentiation from the other European Ixodes, scale bar 200 μm.

closest to those belonging to genogroup A were also documented in Spain and Portugal [12, 14]. In the latter study, 12S and 16S rRNA genes have been targeted in 48 questing *I. ventalloi* (nymphs and adults), resulting in the identification of six haplotypes (IvH1-H6) but with a low degree of nucleotide variation placing them all in Latrofa's genogroup A [12]. **Figure 2** represents the phylogenetic distance, based on 16S rRNA sequences, of the *I. ventalloi* specimens collected in Italy, Spain, and Portugal, comparing to those related (>91% homology) *Ixodes* species. These results highlight the need for further genetic characterization of *I. ventalloi* population, increasing both the molecular coverage and the number of studied specimens from other geographical origins.

The *I. ventalloi* sequences obtained in the aforementioned studies were deposited in GenBank under the accession numbers: KU178964-KU178979 for *cox1*; KU178956-KU178963, KY231931, MF370642-43, MF621228, MF621233, MG210719-20 for 16S rDNA; MF370631-32, MF621221, MF621226, MG210717-18 for 12S rDNA.

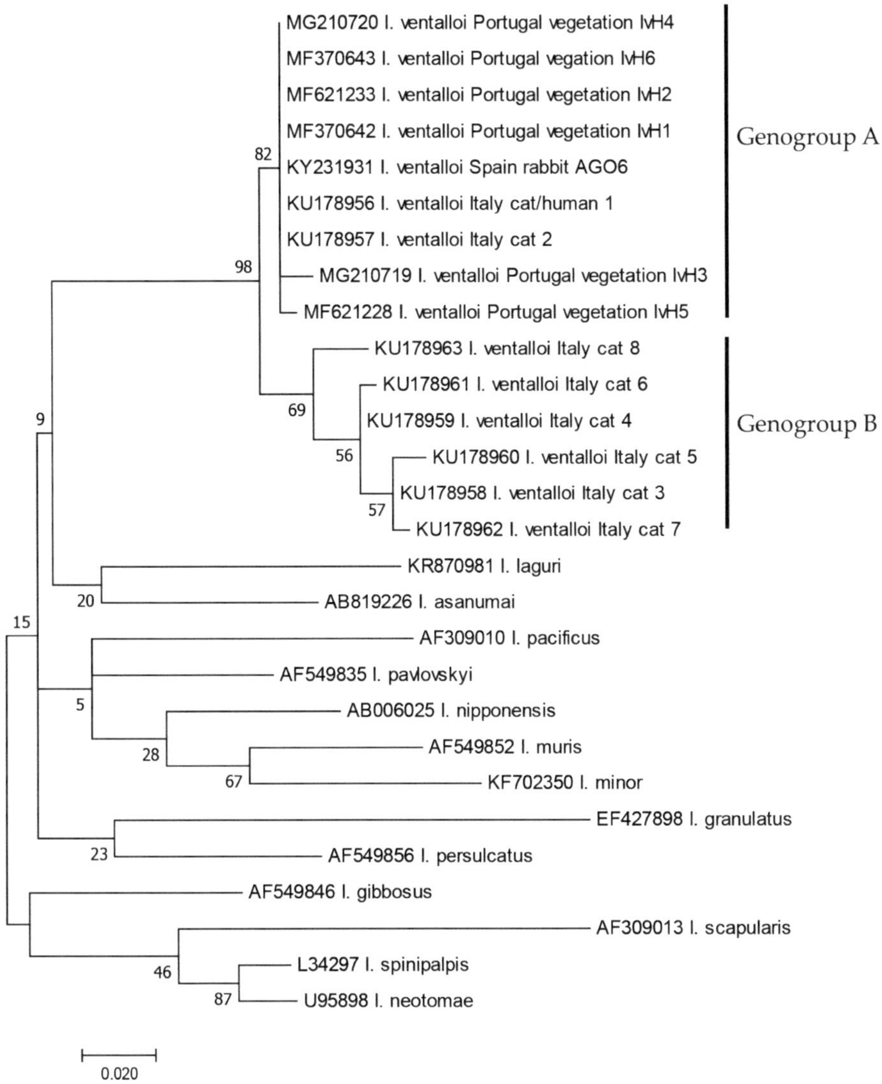

Figure 2.

Phylogenetic trees based on 16S rRNA sequences obtained from Ixodes ventalloi collected in Italy, Spain and Portugal, comparing to sequences of other related (>91% homology) Ixodes species available in GenBank. Phylogenetic relationships were assessed computing the maximum likelihood method on MEGA7 [22]. Best fitting substitution models were determined using MEGA7 model selection method. Phylogenetic tree was constructed using General time reversible model, modulated by using a discrete Gamma distribution (+G) and based on the analysis of 1000 replicates. All positions with less than 75% site coverage were eliminated. That is, fewer than 25% alignment gaps, missing data, and ambiguous bases were allowed at any position. There were a total of 247 positions in the final dataset. Accession numbers are followed by species name, and in some case the origin of sequences and haplotypes designation. Branch lengths represent the number of substitutions per site inferred according to the scale-bar.

3. The permissive "rabbit-tick"

The geographical distribution of *I. ventalloi* includes areas of western Mediterranean Europe (Portugal, Spain, Southern France, Central and Southern Italy, and Cyprus) and Northern Africa (Marroco and Tunisia) [14, 21]. This tick species was also documented in Great Britain (Channel Islands, Lundy Island, and Isles of Scilly) and in southwest Germany, probably as the result of introductions,

Host order and species	Tick stage/sex	Country (or region)	References
Birds			
Strigiformes			
Asio flammeus	F, M, N	Portugal	[9]
Asio otus	F	Great Britain	[16][a], [27]
Athene noctua	F	Spain,	[15]
Tyto alba	N	Portugal	[11]
Galliformes			
Alectoris chukar	ND	Cyprus	[31]
Alectoris rufa	F(+)	France, Italy	[16][b], [32]
Phasianus colchicus	F(+)	France, Italy, North Africa	[16][c], [32]
Passeriformes			
Pica pica	F	France	[16][b]
Turdus merula	N	Great Britain, Portugal	[23, 33]
Turdus pilaris	F	France	[16][b]
Gruiformes			
Rallus aquaticus	ND	Italy	[32]
Mammals			
Lagomorpha			
Lepus europaeus	F(+)	Cyprus, other European regions	[16][e], [31]
Oryctolagus cuniculus	F, M, N, L	France, Great Britain, Portugal, Spain, Morocco, North Africa	[7], [16][d][17, 18], [26][i], [23, 27–30]
Rodentia			
Apodemus sylvaticus	Im	Morocco	[26][i]
Eliomys quercinus	F, N, L	Morocco, Portugal	[7], [26][i]
Gerbillus campestris	Im	Morocco	[26][i]
Hystrix cristata	ND	Italy	[34]
Lemniscomys barbarus	Im	Morocco	[26][i]
Mus spretus	F, N, L	Morocco, Portugal	[7], [26][i]
Rattus rattus	Im	Morocco	[26][i]
Rattus norvegicus	N	Portugal	[11]
Sciurus vulgaris	F	Northern Africa	[16][f]
Eulipotyphla			
Crocidura russula	N	Portugal	[7]
Erinaceus europaeus	F, M, N	Portugal, Spain and North Africa	[6], [16][f], [35]
Carnivora			
Canis familiaris	F	Portugal	[11]
Felis catus	F, M, N	France, Great Britain, Italy, Portugal, North Africa	[8, 10, 11, 13], [16][h], [27, 32, 36], [37]
Genetta genetta	F, M	Spain, other European regions	[16][g], [38]
Herpestes ichneumon	F, M	Spain	[38, 39]

Host order and species	Tick stage/sex	Country (or region)	References
Lynx pardinus	F, M	Spain	[38, 39]
Carnivora			
Martes foina	F	France	[16][b]
Meles meles	F	France	[16][b]
Mustela nivalis	F, M, N, L	Portugal	[7, 11]
Mustela n. numidica	Im	Morocco	[26][i]
Vulpes vulpes	F, M, Im	Cyprus, Morocco Portugal, Spain	[6], [26][i], [31, 38–40]
Primata			
Homo sapiens	F(+)	France, Italy, Portugal	[16][b], [41–44]
Reptiles			
Squamata			
Agama impalearis	Im	Morocco	[26][i]
Chalcides polylepis	Im	Morocco	[26][i]
Eumeces algeriensis	Im	Morocco	[26][i]
Psammodromus algirus	Im	Morocco	[26][i]

ND—No detail is provided regarding sex/stage of the collected tick(s); Im—Immature(s) stage(s) not detailed; F—Female(s); F(+)—Female(s) and possible other specimens as information regarding sex/stage is not detailed in all references; M—Male(s); N—Nymph(s); L—Larva(e).

[a–h]In Gilot and Perez [16], the country or geographical regions was deduced based on the authors' descriptions of the origin of I. ventalloi specimens. [a]Thompson collection. [b]Gilot collection. [c]Gilot and Morel collection. [d]Gilot, Morel, Institute Pasteur and Clifford collections. [e]Institute Pasteur collection. [f]Morel collection. [g]Neumann collection. [h]Gilot, Morel and Thompson collections.

[i]Bailly-Choumara et al. [26] list of the Moroccan host is used with reservations since it was published prior to the differentiation of I. ventalloi from I. festai. In any case, the authors were aware about the synonymy of I. ventalloi and I. festai sensu Arthur. Moreover, I. festai is also listed but placed apart from I. ventalloi.

Table 1.
List of vertebrate species found with Ixodes ventalloi ticks.

but the establishment of *I. ventalloi* populations was only confirmed in the Britain islands [23, 24]. In Portugal, *I. ventalloi* was first identified in 1985, and since then, it has been described across the country mainly in littoral mainland areas and along with other moisture-demanding ticks, such as *Haemaphysalis* spp., *Ixodes frontalis, I. ricinus* [6–8, 10–12, 25].

I. ventalloi is regarded as a three-host, endophilic, and monotropic tick. All development stages are commonly found parasitizing *Oryctolagus cuniculus* and associated to lagomorph's environment; thus, it is popularly designated as the "rabbit-tick" [7, 16–18, 23, 25–30]. However, the list of vertebrate hosts parasitized by *I. ventalloi* is much more broader, including several species of rodents and other small mammals, medium-size carnivores, and occasionally ground-dwelling birds and birds of prey [6–11, 13, 15, 16, 23, 26, 27, 31–43]. **Table 1** resumes the host species that have been documented with *I. ventalloi* ticks. Close to 40 species are so far listed revealing the permissive feeding behavior of this tick, which is not restricted to wild animals. In fact, *I. ventalloi* were found feeding on humans and companion animals, mostly cats and sporadically dogs, as shown in **Table 1**. Regarding cats, the first record of this tick-host association date back to the description of *I. thompsoni* (synonym of *I. ventalloi*) from the material collected in Lundy Island by Thompson [16]. Since then, *I. ventalloi* has been recurrently found feeding on cats in almost all areas where it occurs and in some cases described as the predominant tick species found on this host [8, 10, 11, 13, 27, 32, 36, 37]. Cat parasitism by *I. ventalloi* might be explained by the host free-roaming and hunting habits that place them in close contact with the ground and low vegetation when ambushing small animals. Although *I. ventalloi* is regarded as having a limited potential for dispersal, it can be found actively seeking for hosts at the ground level. This was proven by us in previous studies, when dragging vegetation and grassy ground resulted in the collection of 175 questing *I. ventalloi*, including nymphs, males and females [8–12]. The same result was recently obtained by Torina et al. [45] that have collected 1425 questing *I. ventalloi*, including all tick stages, by dragging vegetation in Palermo's areas during a 2-year study.

The particular association of cats to *I. ventalloi* may contribute to bring this tick to domestic environments and to promote human exposure. In fact, *I. ventalloi* has long been listed as a human-biting tick [16, 41]. In Portugal, the authors recorded the first case of human parasitism by this species in 2014, on behalf of the Surveillance Network for Vectors and Vector-borne Diseases (REVIVE), and keep documenting it every year since then [44, 46]. Although *I. ventalloi* represents a small percentage (less than 1%) of the species found feeding on humans, it is under the scope for potential infections by human pathogens [44, 46]. The increasing number of agents associated to this species in recent years brought back the question regarding the *I. ventalloi* public health relevance.

4. A vector's potential neglected or negligible?

During several years, information regarding *I. ventalloi* pathobiome was almost absent. The first association of this tick to a potential tick-borne agent was reported in 1984 by Chastel et al. [47]. In this study, strains of the coltivirus Eyach (EYAV), a virus belonging to Colorado tick fever group, were isolated from both *I. ventalloi* and *I. ricinus* ticks that were found parasitizing a wild rabbit in Northwestern France. Eyach virus was previously described in *I. ricinus* from West Germany, subsequently found on several wild mammals and indirectly linked to patients with neurological disorders, as tick-borne encephalitis, polyradiculoneuritis, and meningopolyneuritis, on a base of serology [48]. In 2004, we have also reported *I. ventalloi* infection by *Anaplasma phagocytophilum*, a species with variant strains implicated in human and domestic animal cases of granulocytic anaplasmosis [8]. The growing interest on *I. ventalloi* observed in the last 10 years has resulted in an increasing number of papers and the detection of diverse microorganisms associated to this tick species. **Table 2** resumes the microbial agents that have been found in *I. ventalloi*, providing information on ticks stage, sex, and molecular identification (haplotypes), when available. Overall, 13 agents have already been associated to *I. ventalloi,* and infected ticks were found feeding on wild animals, as well as on domestic cats and on a human, pointing for a potential role as vector that might have both medical and veterinary implications.

Another justification for the presence of agent's nucleic acids in parasitizing ticks can also be the presence of host-infected blood in arthropods′ midgut rather than a true vector potential. However, it is worthy of note that some of the *I. ventalloi* positives were indeed unfed ticks, as detailed. The first record dates back to 2004 when the authors were investigating *A. phagocytophilum* in *I. ricinus* and their sympatric ticks in Setubal District, Portugal [8]. The screened sites were mainly suburban wooded areas in some cases used for grazing and with evidence

Microorganism	Ticks origin	Ticks haplotypes§	Reference
Virus			
Coltivirus Eyach	*Oryctolagus cuniculus*	ND	[47]
Bacteria			
Anaplasma marginale	Vegetation	ND	[49]
A. phagocytophilum	Vegetation, *Felis catus*	ND	[8, 10]
	Vegetation	IvH1, IvH3, IvH5	[12]
Ehrlichia canis	*Felis catus*	ND	[36]
Ca Neoehrlichia sp.	Vegetation	ND	[12]
Rickettsia helvetica	*Asio flammeus*	ND	[9]
	Lynx pardinus, *Vulpes vulpes*	ND	[38]
	Felis catus, *Rallus aquaticus*	ND	[32]
	*Felis catus**	ND	[36]
	Homo sapiens	Haplotype 1	[13, 37]
R. monacensis	*Oryctolagus cuniculus*	ND	[29]
	Lynx pardinus, *Vulpes vulpes*, *Genetta genetta*	ND	[38]
	*Felis catus**	ND	[32, 36]
Coxiella burnetii	*Alectoris chukar*, *Lepus europaeus*	ND	[31]
	Vegetation	IvH2, IvH3, IvH5, IvH6	[12]
Bartonella clarridgeiae	*Felis catus*‡	ND	[36]
Borrelia valaisiana	*Felis catus*, *Rallus aquaticus*, *Phasianus colchicus*¥	ND	[32]
B. spielmanii	*Felis catus*, *Phasianus colchicus*¥	ND	[32]
Protozoa			
Leishmania infantum	*Felis catus*‡	ND	[36]
Theileria annulata	Vegetation	ND	[49]

**One tick co-infected with Rickettsia helvetica and R. monacensis [36].*

‡One female tick coinfected with Bartonella clarridgeiae and Leishmania infantum.

¥One tick co-infected with Borrelia valaisiana and B. spielmanii.

§All these haplotypes have been identified as belonging to genogroup A and were submitted to Genbank under the accession numbers: Haplotype 1, KU178956 (16S rDNA) and KU178964 (cox1); IvH1, MF370631 (12S rDNA) and MF370642 (16S rDNA); IvH2, MF621226 (12S rDNA) and MF621233 (16S rDNA); IvH3, MG210717 (12S rDNA) and MG210719 (16S rDNA); IvH5, MF621221 (12S rDNA) and MF621228 (16S rDNA); IvH6, MF370632 (12S rDNA) and MF370643 (16S rDNA), as previously described [12, 13].

Table 2.
List of microorganisms and parasites found in Ixodes ventalloi.

of wild animals presence, as rabbits. Out of the 93 *I. ventalloi* collected, *A. phagocytophilum* was recorded in a questing nymph and also in a male found attached to a free-roaming cat. The sequences obtained from both ticks were found to be a new *A. phagocytophilum* variant based on *groEL* and *msp2* gene analysis [8]. This finding was subsequently reinforced by the detection of the same *A. phagocytophilum* variant also in an *I. ventalloi* female feeding on a cat from another district of mainland, Santarém District [10]. More recently, a retrospective study using the DNA material stored from Setúbal district ticks also resulted in the detection of questing *I. ventalloi* specimens of *Anaplasma marginale* (four nymphs and one male) and *Theileria annulata* (one female) [49]. New data that link more agents to questing *I. ventalloi* were submitted for publication in the beginning of 2018 [12]. That study was undertaken in Parque Florestal de Monsanto (PFM), a recreational area located in the urban perimeter of Lisbon city. This is a highly used park for petting and several outdoor activities. Overall, eight tick species were found questing in PFM with a preponderance of *I. ventalloi*. A preliminary 1-year screening to define the best season for collection, established that the period of activity for this species extended from November to June, with a peak in spring (**Figure 3**) [50]. Interesting, both of these findings (abundance and seasonality) were reinforced in Torina et al. comprehensive study [45]. In our case, the diversity of PFM ticks and the particular abundance of *I. ventalloi* were attributed to the park's wild population, composed of over 100 species of small mammals and birds [51].

Regarding tick-borne agents, questing *I. ventalloi* in PFM were found harboring *A. phagocytophilum* (two males, one female, and two nymphs), *Coxiella burnetii* (five males, three females, and one nymph), and a potentially new agent

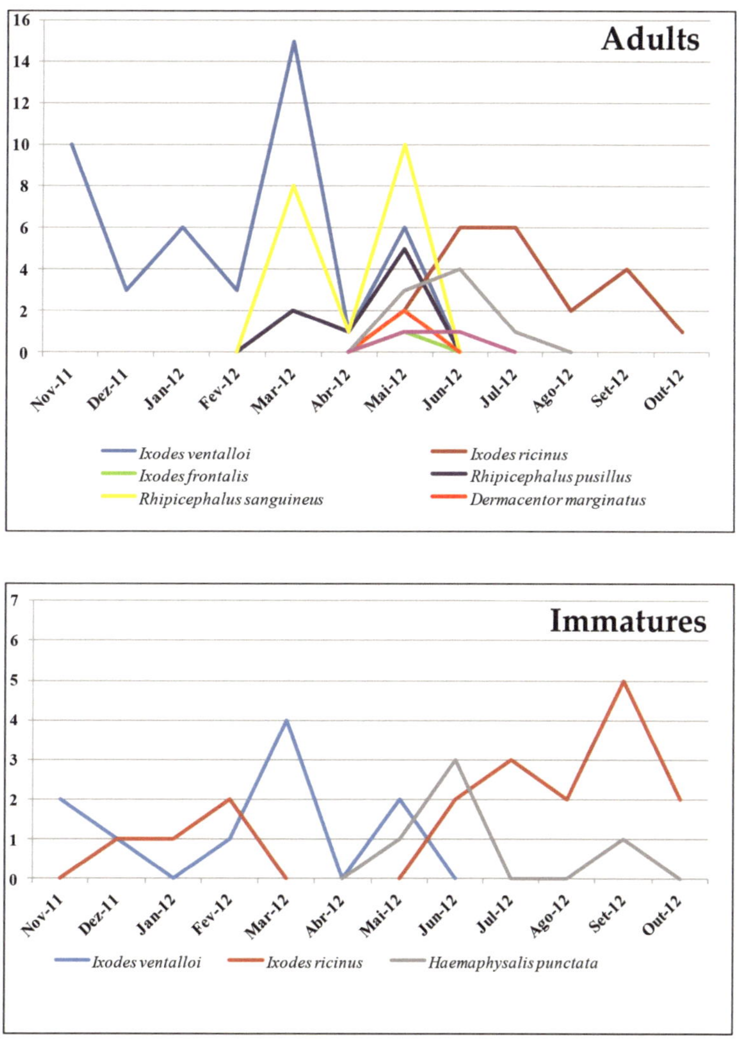

Figure 3.
The distribution of immature and adult tick species collected in PFM during 1-year period (2011–2012) [50].

close related to *Candidatus* (*Ca.*) Neoehrlichia mikurensis (one female and one male). Interestingly, two *A. phagocytophilum* variants were detected [12]. The more representative was a new variant of *A. phagocytophilum* previously detected in both Setúbal and Santarém districts (and here found on four ticks) [8, 10]. This reinforces previous data sustaining a divergent variant of *A. phagocytophilum*, not clustering in none of the four ecotypes defined by Jahfari et al. [52], with the closest sequence sharing only 95% homology and belonging to ecotype IV that is composed of sequences of the agent derived from birds. Another *A. phagocytophilum* variant was obtained from a single *I. ventalloi*, clustering the ecotype I that is composed by agent's sequences associated to human and domestic animal cases of granulocytic anaplasmosis [52]. It was also worth of mention that positive ticks were found questing in different occasions showing the existence of active cycles for these agents in PFM [12]. The molecular identification of nine positive ticks confirmed that all belonged to Latrofa's genotype A, based on 16S rDNA analysis. The obtained haplotypes and the GenBank accession numbers are presented in **Table 2**.

In all the aforementioned Portuguese areas, infected *I. ventalloi* were found questing along with other moisture-demanding ticks, as the mega-vector *I. ricinus*. Both tick species are considered sympatric sharing geographical distribution, vertebrate hosts, and possible their agents [11]. The presence of alternate ticks (generally endophilic ticks) has been associated to the existence of secondary maintenance cycles for some *Ixodes*-borne agents [53]. If *I. ventalloi* has such a role and thus contributes indirectly to the occurrence of *I. ricinus*-borne diseases is yet to be investigated.

5. Conclusion

I. ventalloi has been relegated to the sidelines for years due to its endophilic nature, apparent host specificity, and unknown vector importance. Accumulated evidence is, however, revealing a different reality for this small *Ixodes*. As revised here, *I. ventalloi* presents a permissive feeding behaviors that might promote exposure to several blood-borne pathogens and the list of agents found in this species keeps growing. Of note is the fact that *I. ventalloi* is broadly found feeding on cats and can also parasitize men. Moreover, it is sympatric to the mega-vector *I. ricinus* and might contribute to the maintenance of its agents. Altogether these suggest a vector role for *I. ventalloi*, either directly or by sympatry with other ticks species, with potential public health implications and deserving further investigation.

Acknowledgements

This work was supported by the FCT project PTDC/SAU-PAR/28947/2017. The authors thank Miguel Flores for the library assistance.

Conflict of interest

The authors do not disclose any conflict of interest.

Author details

Ana Sofia Santos* and Maria Margarida Santos-Silva
Center for Vectors and Infectious Disease Research (CEVDI), National Institute of Health Doutor Ricardo Jorge, Águas de Moura, Portugal

*Address all correspondence to: ana.santos@insa.min-saude.pt

References

[1] Balashov YS. Bloodsucking ticks (Ixodoidea): Vectors of diseases of man and animals. Vol. 8. Miscellaneous Publications of the Entomological Society of America. Baltimore: Entomological Society of America; 1968. pp. 1-376

[2] Krantz GW. A Manual of Acarology. 2nd ed. Corvallis: Oregon State University Book Stores; 1978

[3] Sonenshine DE, Roe RM. Overview ticks, people, and animals. In: Sonenshine DE, Roe RM, editors. Biology of Ticks. 2nd ed. Vol. 1. New York: Oxford University Press; 2014. pp. 3-16

[4] Estrada-Peña A, Mans BJ. Tick-induced paralysis and toxicoses. In: Sonenshine DE, Roe EM, editors. Biology of Ticks. 2nd ed. Vol. 2. New York: Oxford University Press; 2014. pp. 313-332

[5] Guglielmone AA, Robbins RG, Apanaskevich DA, Petney TN, Estrada-Peña A, Horak IG. Ticks feeding on humans. In: Guglielmone AA, Robbins RG, Apanaskevich DA, Petney TN, Estrada-Peña A, Horak IG, editors. Hard Ticks of the World: (Acari: Ixodida: Ixodidae). Netherlands: Springer Science+Business Media Dordrecht; 2014. pp. 715-716. DOI: 10.1007/978-94-007-7497-1

[6] Dias JATS. Um novo Ixodídeo (Acarina, Ixodoidea) para a fauna de Portugal. *Ixodes ventalloi* Gil Collado, 1936. Actas do II Congresso Ibérico de Entomologia. Boletim da Sociedade Portuguesa de Entomologia. 1985;**4**(Supl I):149-158

[7] Dias JATS, Santos-Reis M. A carraça *Ixodes ventalloi* Gil Collado, 1936 como principal ectoparasita de uma população de doninhas (*Mustela nivalis* Linnaeus, 1766) em Portugal. Garcia de Orta: Série de Zoologia. 1989;**14**:35-50

[8] Santos AS, Santos-Silva MM, Almeida VC, Bacellar F, Dumler JS. Detection of *Anaplasma phagocytophilum* DNA in *Ixodes* ticks (Acari: Ixodidae) from Madeira Island and Setúbal District, mainland Portugal. Emerging Infectious Diseases. 2004;**10**(9):1643-1648

[9] Santos-Silva MM, Sousa R, Santos AS, Melo P, Encarnação V, Bacellar F. Ticks parasitizing wild birds in Portugal: detection of *Rickettsia aeschlimannii*, *R. helvetica* and *R. massiliae*. Experimental and Applied Acarology. 2006;**39**:331-338. DOI: 10.1007/s10493-006-9008-3

[10] Santos AS, Santos-Silva MM, Sousa R, Bacellar F, Dumler JS. PCR-based survey of *Anaplasma phagocytophilum* in Portuguese ticks (Acari: Ixodidae). Vector Borne and Zoonotic Diseases. 2009 Feb;**9**(1):33-40. DOI: 10.1089/vbz.2008.0051

[11] Santos-Silva MM, Beati L, Santos AS, De Sousa R, Núncio MS, Melo P, et al. The hard-tick fauna of mainland Portugal (Acari: Ixodidae): An update on geographical distribution and known associations with hosts pathogens. Experimental and Applied Acarology. 2011;**55**(1):85-121. DOI: 10.1007/s10493-011-9440-x

[12] Santos AS, de Bruin A, Veloso AR, Marques C, Pereira da Fonseca I, de Sousa I, et al. Detection of *Anaplasma phagocytophilum*, *Candidatus* Neoehrlichia sp., *Coxiella burnetii*, and *Rickettsia* spp. in questing ticks from a recreational park, Portugal. Tick and Tick-Borne Diseases. 2018;**9**(6):1555-1564. DOI: 10.1016/j.ttbdis.2018.07.010

[13] Latrofa MS, Giannelli A, Persichetti MF, Pennisi MG, Solano-Gallego L, Brianti E, et al. *Ixodes ventalloi*: Morphological and molecular support for species integrity. Parasitology

Research. 2017;**116**(1):251-258. DOI: 10.1007/s00436-016-5286-9

[14] Estrada-Peña A, Venzal JM, Nava S. Redescription, molecular features, and neotype deposition of *Rhipicephalus pusillus* Gil Collado and *Ixodes ventalloi* Gil Collado (Acari, Ixodidae). Zootaxa. 2018;**4442**(2):262-276. DOI: 10.11646/zootaxa.4442.2.4

[15] Gil Collado J. Acaros Ixodoideos de Cataluña y Baleares. Treballs del Museu de Ciencies Naturals de Barcelona, Serie Entomologica. 1936;**11**(2):1-8

[16] Gilot B, Perez C. Individualisation et caractérisation de deux *Ixodes* actuelement confondus: *I. festai* Rondelli, 1926, *I. ventalloi* Gil Collado, 1936 (Acarina, Ixodoidea). Revue Suisse de Zoologie. 1978;**85**(1):143-149

[17] Morel PC, Perez C. Morphologie des stages preimaginales des ixodoidea s. str. d'Europe occidentale. V – Les larves des *Ixodes* s. str. Acarologia. 1977;**19**(3):395-402

[18] Morel PC, Perez C. Morphologie des stages preimaginales des ixodoidea s. str. dÉurope occidentale. V – Les nymphs des *Ixodes* s. str. Acarologia. 1977;**19**(4):579-586

[19] Gil Collado J, Guillen Llera J, Zapateiro Ramos LM. Clave para la Identificacion de los Ixodoidea Españoles (Adultos). Revista Ibérica de Parasitologia. 1979;**39**:107-118

[20] Gil Collado J, Sanchez-Covisa A, Rodrigues Rodriguez JÁ. Detalles ultraestructurales de *Ixodes ventalloi*, Gil Collado 1936 (Acarina: Metastigmata). Proceedings of the VI Congreso Nacional de Parasitología y I Congresso Ibérico de Parasitología, Cáceres: In; 1989

[21] Pérez-Eid C. *Ixodes* (*Ixodes*) *ventalloi* Gil Collado, 1936. In: Pérez-Eid C, editor. Les tiques. Identification, biologie importance médicale et vétérinaire. Monographies de microbiologie. Paris: TEC & DOC Lavoisier; 2007. pp. 124-127

[22] Kumar S, Stecher G, Tamura K. MEGA7: Molecular Evolutionary Genetics Analysis version 7.0 for bigger datasets. Molecular Biology and Evolution. 2016;**33**:1870-1874. DOI: 10.1093/molbev/msw054

[23] Jameson LJ, Medlock JM. Tick surveillance in Great Britain. Vector Borne and Zoonotic Diseases. 2011;**11**(4):403-412. DOI: 10.1089/vbz.2010.0079

[24] Petney TN, Pfäffle MP, Skuballa JD. An annotated checklist of the ticks (Acari: Ixodida) of Germany. Systematic and Applied Acarology. 2012;**17**(2):115-170

[25] Petney TN, Otranto D, Dantas-Torres F, Pfäffle MP. Ixodes ventalloi Gil Collado, 1936. In: Estrada-Peña A, Mihalca AD, Petney, editors. Ticks of Europe and North Africa. A Guide to Species Identification. Switzerland: Springer International Publishing; 2017. pp. 183-187. DOI: 10.1007/978-3-319-63760-0

[26] Bailly-Choumara H, Morel PC, Rageau J. Sommaire des donnes actuelles sur les tiques du Maroc (Acari, Ixodoidea). Le Bulletin de l'Institut Scientifique. 1976;**1**:101-117

[27] Martin KP. Provisional Atlas of the Ticks (Ixodoidea) of the British Isles. Biological Recods Center, Institute of Terrestrial Ecology Monks Wood Experimental Station, Dorchester, Great Britain: Henry Ling Ltd at the Dorset Press; 1988. p. 62

[28] Marquez FJ, Guiguen C. Distribution sur l'hote des ixodoides parasites d'*Oryctolagus cuniculus* (L.) et facteurs qui l'affectent. Acarologia. 1992;**23**:141-148

[29] Márquez FJ. Spotted fever group *Rickettsia* in ticks from southeastern Spain natural parks. Experimental and Applied Acarology. 2008;**45**(3-4):185-194. DOI: 10.1007/s10493-008-9181-7

[30] González J, Valcárcel F, Pérez-Sánchez JL, Tercero-Jaime JM, Olmeda AS. Seasonal dynamics of ixodid ticks on wild rabbits *Oryctolagus cuniculus* (Leporidae) from Central Spain. Experimental and Applied Acarology. 2016;**70**(3):369-380. DOI: 10.1007/s10493-016-0069-7

[31] Psaroulaki A, Chochlakis D, Angelakis E, Ioannou I, Tselentis Y. *Coxiella burnetii* in wildlife and ticks in an endemic area. Transactions of the Royal Society of Tropical Medicine and Hygiene. 2014;**108**(10):625-631. DOI: 10.1093/trstmh/tru134

[32] Tomassone L, Grego E, Auricchio D, Iori A, Giannini F, Rambozzi L. Lyme borreliosis spirochetes and spotted fever group rickettsiae in ixodid ticks from Pianosa Island, Tuscany Archipelago, Italy. Vector Borne and Zoonotic Diseases. 2013;**13**(2):84-91. DOI: 10.1089/vbz.2012.1046

[33] Norte AC, da Silva LP, Tenreiro PJ, Felgueiras MS, Araújo PM, Lopes PB, et al. Patterns of tick infestation and their *Borrelia burgdorferi* s.l. infection in wild birds in Portugal. Ticks and Tick-borne Diseases. 2015;**6**(6):743-750. DOI: 10.1016/j.ttbdis.2015.06.010

[34] Mori E, Sforzi A, Menchetti M, Mazza G, Lovari S, Pisanu B. Ectoparasite load in the crested porcupine *Hystrix cristata* Linnaeus, 1758 in Central Italy. Parasitology Research. 2015;**114**(6):2223-2229. DOI: 10.1007/s00436-015-4413-3

[35] Domínguez G. Ectoparásitos de los mamíferos silvestres del norte de Burgos (España). Galemys. 2003;**15**(1):47-60

[36] Pennisi MG, Persichetti MF, Serrano L, Altet L, Reale S, Gulotta L, et al. Ticks and associated pathogens collected from cats in Sicily and Calabria (Italy). Parasites & Vectors. 2015;**8**:512. DOI: 10.1186/s13071-015-1128-3

[37] Otranto D, Dantas-Torres F, Napoli E, Solari Basano F, Deuster K, Pollmeier M, et al. Season-long control of flea and tick infestations in a population of cats in the Aeolian archipelago using a collar containing 10% imidacloprid and 4.5% flumethrin. Veterinary Parasitology. 2017;**248**:80-83. DOI: 10.1016/j.vetpar.2017.10.023

[38] Márquez FJ, Millán J. Rickettsiae in ticks from wild and domestic carnivores of Doñana National Park (Spain) and surrounding area. Clinical Microbiology and Infection. 2009;**15**(Suppl 2):224-226. DOI: 10.1111/j.1469-0691.2008.02147.x

[39] Millán J, Ruiz-Fons F, Márquez FJ, Viota M, López-Bao JV, Paz Martín-Mateo M. Ectoparasites of the endangered Iberian lynx *Lynx pardinus* and sympatric wild and domestic carnivores in Spain. Medical and Veterinary Entomology. 2007;**21**(3):248-254

[40] Martínez-Carrasco C, Ruiz de Ybáñez MR, Sagarminaga JL, Garijo MM, Moreno F, Acosta I, et al. Parasites of the red fox (*Vulpes vulpes* Linnaeus, 1758) in Murcia, southeast Spain. Revue de Médecine Vétérinaire. 2007;**158**(7):331-335

[41] Gilot B, Marjolet M. Contribution à l'étude du parasitisme humain par les tiques (Ixodidae et Argasidae), plus particulièrement dans le sud-est de la France. Médecine et Maladies Infectieuses. 1982;**12**(6):340-351

[42] Sanogo YO, Parola P, Shpynov S, Camicas JL, Brouqui P, Caruso G, et al. Genetic diversity of bacterial agents detected in ticks removed from

asymptomatic patients in northeastern Italy. Annals of the New York Academy of Sciences. 2003;**990**:182-190

[43] Otranto D, Dantas-Torres F, Giannelli A, Latrofa MS, Cascio A, Cazzin S, et al. Ticks infesting humans in Italy and associated pathogens. Parasites & Vectors. 2014;7:328

[44] Santos-Silva MM, Lopes de Carvalho I, Santos AS, Núncio S, Sousa R, Equipa REVIVE. Estudo dos ixodídeos removidos de humanos no âmbito do programa REVIVE, 2011-2015. Boletim Epidemiológico Observações. 2017;**18**(2):10-13

[45] Torina A, Blanda V, Blanda M, Auteri M, La Russa F, Scimeca S, et al. A geographical information system based approach for integrated strategies of tick surveillance and control in the peri-urban natural reserve of Monte Pellegrino (Palermo, Southern Italy). International Journal of Environmental Research and Public Health. 2018;**15**:404. DOI: 10.3390/ijerph15030404

[46] Santos AS, Santos-Silva M, Lopes de Carvalho I, Milhano N, Chaínho L, Luz T, et al. REVIVE, a surveillance program on vectors and vector-borne pathogens in Portugal—Four years experience on ticks. In: Abstract Book the 2nd Conference on Neglected Vectors and Vector-borne Diseases; 31 March-2 April 2015; Izmir, Turquia. pp. 39-40

[47] Chastel C, Main AJ, Couatarmanac'h A, Le Lay G, Knudson DL, Quillien MC, et al. Isolation of Eyach vírus (Reoviridae, Colorado tick fever group) from *Ixodes ricinus* and *I. ventalloi* ticks in France. Archives of Virology. 1984;**82**(3-4):161-171

[48] Attoui H, Mohd Jaafar F, de Micco P, de Lamballerie X. Coltiviruses and seadornaviruses in North America, Europe, and Asia. Emerging Infectious Diseases. 2005;**11**(11):1673-1679

[49] Antunes S, Ferrolho J, Domingues N, Santos AS, Santos-Silva MM, Domingos A. *Anaplasma marginale* and *Theileria annulata* in questing ticks from Portugal. Experimental and Applied Acarology. 2016;**70**(1):79-88. DOI: 10.1007/s10493-016-0057-y

[50] Veloso AR. Pesquisa de Coxiella burnetii em ixodídeos capturados em parques urbanos de Lisboa [thesis]. Lisboa: Faculdade de Medicina Veterinária, Universidade Técnica de Lisboa; 2013

[51] Biodiversidade: Biodiversidade na Cidade de Lisboa: Uma estatégia para 2020 [Internet]. 2015. Available from: http://www.cm-lisboa.pt/fileadmin/VIVER/Ambiente/Biodiversidade/Estudos/Biodiversidade.pdf [Accessed: May 29, 2018]

[52] Jahfari S, Coipan EC, Fonville M, van Leeuwen AD, Hengeveld P, Heylen D, et al. Circulation of four *Anaplasma phagocytophilum* ecotypes in Europe. Parasites & Vectors. 2014;7:365

[53] Bown KJ, Begon M, Bennett M, Woldehiwet Z, Ogden NH. Seasonal dynamics of *Anaplasma phagocytophila* in a rodent-tick (*Ixodes trianguliceps*) system, United Kingdom. Emerging Infectious Disease. 2003;**9**:63-70

Section 3

Vector Borne Zoonotic Diseases and Pathogens

Chapter 4

Sandfly-Borne Viruses of Demonstrated/Relevant Medical Importance

Nazli Ayhan and Remi N. Charrel

Abstract

Sandflies show distribution in a vast geographical area from Europe to Asia, Africa, Australia, and Central and South America where they can transmit a large number of viruses. Between these viruses, the most important are grouped into the *Phlebovirus* genus (family *Phenuiviridae*). Among them, several sandfly-borne phleboviruses cause self-limiting febrile disease (sandfly fever) or central and peripheral nervous system infections. Data concerning the geographic distribution of these phleboviruses has drastically increased during the last decade in both the new and the old worlds. The current situation depicts a high viral diversity with taxonomic groups containing human pathogenic and non-pathogenic viruses. This merits to provide insight to address the question of medical and veterinary public health impact of all these viruses, which are poorly studied. To do so, integrated and translational approaches must use ecological, epidemiological, serological and direct clinical evidence. Beside, other viruses transmitted by sandflies and belonging to *Rhabdoviridae* and *Reoviridae* families can also be of veterinary and public health importance. The chapter aims to provide a comprehensive view of the sandfly-borne viral pathogens of the public health impact on humans and other vertebrates in the old and new worlds.

Keywords: sandfly-borne phleboviruses, sandfly fever, phlebovirus, Toscana virus, Sandfly fever Naples virus, Sandfly fever Sicilian virus, Punta Toro virus, Vesiculovirus, Chandipura virus, Changuinola virus

1. Introduction

Sandflies are present in tropical and subtropical, arid and semi-arid areas and temperate zones including southern Europe, Asia, Africa, Australia, Central and South America. Phlebotomine sandflies are tiny diptera insects grouped in the family Psychodidae, subfamily Phlebotominae. To date, over 800 species are estimated to exist in different regions of the world [1]. Two genera (*Phlebotomus* and *Sergentomyia*) of Phlebotominae are mostly recorded in the old world (OW) and the other genus *Lutzomyia* exists in the new world (NW) [2]. Only females are hematophagous and require a blood meal to develop their eggs. Sandflies take blood from a wide range of animals such as cold-blooded vertebrates, mammals and birds; trophic preferences vary depending on the sandfly species.

Of the 800 sandfly species, at least 98 are proven or suspected vectors of microorganisms capable to cause parasitic, viral or bacterial diseases in vertebrates [1].

This chapter will focus essentially on sandfly-borne viruses, which have been proven agents of diseases in humans.

The arthropod-borne diseases including sandfly-borne viral diseases affect urban, peri-urban, and rural population but mostly the communities with poor living conditions. Economic, social and ecological conditions have a huge impact on sandfly-borne viral diseases [3, 4]. The factors that described as associated with arthropod-borne diseases emergence or invasion are (i) competent vector and vertebrate host population repeatedly in contact within an appropriate environment, (ii) vertebrate or vector host species composition changes, (iii) environmental or niche changes and (iv) genetic changes [5].

Although sandflies can transmit a number of arthropod-borne viruses within the families *Phenuiviridae*, *Reoviridae* and *Rhabdoviridae*, they remain neglected vectors of viral diseases in contrast with a high interest for parasitic diseases such as leishmaniasis. The three virus families contain human/animal pathogens. In the *Rhabdoviridae* family, attention will be given to Chandipura virus; in the *Reoviridae* family, we will focus on Changuinola virus [2, 6–8]. In the *Phenuiviridae* family, we will focus on Sandfly fever Sicilian virus, Sandfly fever Naples virus, Toscana virus, Adria virus and Punta Toro virus (PTV).

2. Sandfly-borne phleboviruses

Phleboviruses are enveloped viruses with single-stranded trisegmented RNA. They contain three genomics segments: L (Large) segment encodes the viral RNA polymerase (RdRp), M (medium) segment encodes envelope glycoproteins (Gn and Gc) and non-structural protein m (NSm) and S (small) segment encodes nucleocapsid protein (N) and non-structural protein s (NSs) [9].

Currently, 10 species within the genus *Phlebovirus* are recognized by the International Committee on Taxonomy of Viruses (ICTV): *Sandfly fever Naples virus, Salehabad virus, Rift Valley fever virus, Uukuniemi virus, Bujaru virus, Candiru virus, Chilibre virus, Frijoles virus, Punta Toro virus,* and *Severe fever with thrombocytopenia syndrome virus*. Of interest, almost 40 phleboviruses are still listed as tentative species for which the ICTV has not officially ruled; interestingly, Sandfly fever Sicilian virus still belongs to this pending group although discovered in 1943 [10].

Phleboviruses can be detected and isolated from blood-sucking female sandflies and from non-blood-sucking males in equal proportions [11–14]. This suggests that alternative transmission pathways (other than blood-borne from vertebrate reservoir) such as transovarial transmission (female to offsprings) and/or venereal transmission play an important role in the natural cycle [2]. Experimental results done with colonized *P. papatasi* sandflies proved venereal virus transmission and transovarial virus transmission [15]. Viral maintenance during the diapausing period of *Phlebotomus perniciosus* larvae was proved and was not affected by transstadial transmission in laboratory [15]. These routes of virus transmission suggest that phleboviruses can be sustainably transmitted from one generation of sandflies to the next generation. It also raises the question of whether a vertebrate host acting as reservoir is required or not for virus perpetuation. To date, these experiments have been performed primarily with high passage colonies and should be taken with caution because laboratory reared sandflies may behave differently from wild populations. In addition, they have been performed with few species of phlebovirus and with *P. papatasi* and *P. perfiliewi* only. Elucidation of phlebovirus maintenance and transmission is crucial to understand better the natural history of these viruses and to develop adapted method to combat those which are human pathogens [15–17]. Although several sandfly-borne phlebovirus species were isolated from humans, bats and sandflies [18–23], there is no undisputable evidence that vertebrates play an important role in the natural history of sandfly-borne phleboviruses other that as dead-end hosts.

With recently discovered novel viruses, the geographic distribution of phleboviruses has drastically increased in both the new and the old worlds. The current situation depicts a high viral diversity with taxonomic groups containing pathogenic and non-pathogenic viruses. This merits to provide insight to address the question of medical and veterinary public health impact of all these viruses, which are poorly studied.

2.1 Sandfly-borne phleboviruses in the old world

In the old world (OW), the risk for the infection with sandfly-borne phleboviruses is high depending upon the presence and the density of vectors [24].

Historic and recent epidemics have been caused by sandfly-borne phleboviruses in the OW. In 1937, a massive outbreak occurred in, Athens, Greece [25, 26]. During World War II (WWII), outbreaks were described among out-comer soldiers in the Mediterranean basin and Middle East (the Austrian Commission in Balkan countries, British and German troops in the Mediterranean area) [17, 26, 27].

After WWII, sandfly fever epidemics were reported in Belgrade, Serbia, where thousands were sick [28], with subsequent spread into other regions of the Balkans [29–32]. More recently, large epidemics were recorded in Cyprus, Iraq, Turkey and Ethiopia [33–36].

In addition, during the last two decades, an impressive number of novel phleboviruses was either isolated or detected by molecular techniques in France, Italy, Portugal, Greece, Albania, Croatia, Bosnia Herzegovina, Turkey, Iran, Tunisia, Algeria and Morocco [11–14, 23, 37–43]. Accordingly, the Mediterranean area witnesses a very high diversity of phleboviruses transmitted by sandflies [44]. This situation has raised the public health concerns in southern Europe, North Africa and in the Middle East [11, 13, 14, 39, 41, 45, 46].

OW sandfly-borne phleboviruses can be classified into three serological complexes, which are also regarded as taxonomic species, Salehabad species, Sandfly fever Naples species and Sandfly fever Sicilian tentative species.

Sandfly fever Sicilian and Sandfly fever Naples viruses cause fever, also known as "sandfly fever", "Pappataci fever" or "three-day fever". It is not possible to distinguish Sandfly fever Sicilian virus infection from Sandfly fever Naples virus infection based on clinical signs, which are virtually identical. They both cause abrupt illness with fever, headache, malaise, photophobia, myalgia and retro-orbital pain usually lasting 2–3 days after 3–5 day incubation [47].

Toscana virus, which belongs to the *Sandfly fever Naples* species, is so far the most pathogenic sandfly-borne phlebovirus due to its propensity to affect the central nervous system (CNS) and cause meningitis and meningoencephalitis [45]. Recently, Adria virus, identified in a case of meningitis, is the first virus belonging to the *Salehabad* species to display human pathogenesis [38].

2.1.1 Sandfly fever

Before WWII, the knowledge on sandfly fever was limited to clinical and epidemiological grounds. It was known that the fever caused by a filterable agent and transmitted by *Phlebotomus papatasi* sandflies [48, 49]. Early assumptions claimed that sandfly fever might be caused by distinct agents or viruses, despite it was impossible to distinguish them from the clinical symptoms [47, 50].

Between 1934 and 1939, human sera samples from sandfly fever virus-infected individuals (presumably containing the infectious agent) were inoculated into rhesus monkeys which presented with febrile illness [51]. Inoculation of infectious human serum (i) into chick embryos showed lesions on the chorioallantoic membrane, whereas (ii) no clinical sign were noticed after inoculation to guinea pigs, rabbits or dogs [47]. Three out of four human volunteers without a previous sandfly fever history developed the typical symptoms and fever after inoculation of 1 ml of the pool of acute sandfly fever serum [47]. Subsequently, *Phlebotomus papatasi*, *Culex pipiens* and *Pulex irritans* fed on sandfly fever acutely infected volunteers, only *P. papatasi* was able to transmit the disease to naïve volunteers [47]. In 1937, a massive outbreak occurred in Athens, Greece [26]. However, most of the outbreaks occurred in non-native persons having entered the endemic area for the first time recently such as soldiers [13]. During WWII, several outbreaks of sandfly fever knocked down battalions of soldiers in both the Allied and Axis troops which were stationed in the Middle East, the Mediterranean and North Africa [17, 52, 53]. The suspected variety of causing agents was shown through isolation of two different viruses names Naples and Sicilian virus from sick soldiers in southern Italy [47, 53]. The antigenic differences between Naples virus and Sicilian virus were confirmed by human cross-immunity test, neutralization and complement fixation test [54].

2.1.2 Sandfly fever Naples virus

Sandfly fever Naples virus was first isolated from blood of a febrile soldier who became ill when stationed in Naples, Italy in 1944 [47]. Afterward, Naples virus was isolated again (i) from febrile patients in Egypt, Turkmenia, Pakistan, Italy, Cyprus and India [55–61] (ii) and from sandflies in Egypt (*P. papatasi*), in Italy (*P. perniciosus*) and Serbia (*P. perfiliewi*) [19, 59, 62]. This was the first clue that Naples virus could be transmitted by distinct vector species. A large and seminal neutralization-based seroprevalence study, performed by Tesh et al. in 1976, showed that Naples virus was likely to have a much wider distribution than initially believed from virus isolation reports [24]; indeed, neutralizing antibodies were detected in human populations from Bangladesh, Ethiopia, Greece, Iraq, Morocco, Saudi Arabia, Sudan, Djibouti, Turkey and former Yugoslavia [24]. Highest rates (55–62%) were observed in Egypt, former Yugoslavia (now Croatia), and Turkey. Another study reported neutralizing antibodies in populations living in Turkmenia, Tajikistan, Uzbekistan, and Moldavia [63]. Clearly, Naples virus circulation has drastically decreased after the 1980s, and the absence of virus isolation or PCR detection, despite an increasing number of studies conducted in previously endemic areas, question whether Naples virus has gone extinct or not [58].

2.1.2.1 Toscana virus

Toscana virus (TOSV) was first isolated from *P. perniciosus* in central Italy in 1971 [17]. It has taken 12 years to recognize that TOSV was capable to infect humans and was able to cause not only sandfly fever, but also more severe infections characterized by central nervous system (CNS) manifestations such as meningitis and encephalitis. The first cases pointing out that Toscana virus causes CNS infections came from two travelers returning from Italy and Portugal to the United States and Sweden, respectively [64, 65]. This underlines the importance of travel-related medicine in the surveillance of infectious diseases, particularly vector-borne infectious diseases. Most of the Toscana virus case records are coming from important or autochthonous human cases from the Mediterranean basin countries [45, 70]. Autochthonous cases in humans have been reported in Italy [71], Greece [72], Cyprus [73], Croatia [74], Turkey [75, 76], Portugal [77] and France [78]. However, these cases account for a minimal proportion of literature-described cases. In most countries, where TOSV is endemic, it is not a notifiable disease; this together with the absence of pathognomonic clinical sign, and the very limited number of commercially available diagnostic assay may explain why autochthonous cases are drastically under detected, and that most of reported cases have affected travelers, the diagnosis of which is done when returning to their homeland. TOSV cases in travelers have been reported from Italy [66], France [67], Spain [68, 69] and Portugal [64], but also from the Mediterranean islands such as Cyprus [73], Elba [79, 80], Sicily [81] and Sardinia [82].

Seroepidemiological studies showed the presence of neutralizing antibodies against Toscana virus in several Mediterranean countries, however, the rates vary depending on the region Mediterranean basin considered as endemic region of Toscana virus [45, 71, 74, 78, 83–88].

Special attention must also be brought to the technique used for serology, since results can greatly vary due to different levels of cross-reactivity depending on the assay; for instance, the most stringent technique is based on neutralization assays whereas ELISA or immunofluorescence techniques are more prone to cross-reactivity between phleboviruses within the same antigenic group, but also between antigenically distinct phleboviruses [88–90].

The geographic distribution of sandfly-borne phleboviruses can also be measured by surveillance of non-human vertebrates such as domestic animals: such studies have demonstrated that TOSV was actively circulating in Portugal, Greece, Cyprus and Algeria [83–85] from the study of dog sera, and in Kosovo from studying cow and sheep sera [86]. TOSV was also isolated and/or detected in different phlebotomine species such as *P. perniciosus, P. perfiliewi, P. longicuspis, P. sergenti, P. neglectus and Sergentomyia minuta* in Italy, France, Spain, Croatia, Morrocco, Tunisia, Algeria and Corsica [13, 18, 82, 87, 91–96]. These results tend to suggest that TOSV can be transmitted by species other that *P. perniciosus* and *P. perfiliewi*. Such data are compatible with the fact that TOSV might be more widely dispersed than believed from the early studies. Of course, this merit to be further investigated through experimental studies addressing competence of these species for TOSV. TOSV belongs to the *Sandfly fever Naples* species.

To date, three genetic groups of TOSV have been recognized, and they are called lineages A, B and C. Although only one lineage has been identified in a given country, the co-circulation of two lineages has been shown in France, in Turkey, and in Croatia. It is possible that different lineages are transmitted by the same sandfly species and that sympatry may be frequent [91, 93, 97]. Recent Toscana virus antibody characterization assay performed with 41 patients diagnosed with Toscana virus meningitis of meningoencephalitis found that specific IgM titers were high during acute infection up to day 30, the presence of IgM antibodies lasts up to 6 months after acute infection in 71% of cases, however IgG antibodies against Toscana virus persisted at least 2 years in the patients, which gets in line with the fact that TOSV infection is associated with long-term, maybe lifelong immunity [88]. There is accumulating evidence that TOSV is one important cause of meningitis and encephalitis during the warm season and that it should be included in the panel of microorganisms to be systematically tested in clinical microbiology laboratory for patients presenting with febrile illness, CNS and peripheral nervous system manifestations.

2.1.3 Sandfly fever Sicilian virus

Sandfly fever Sicilian virus (SFSV) was first isolated, characterized and named Sicilian virus, from the serum of a US soldier, presenting with sandfly fever when he was stationed in Palerma (Sicily) after the landing of the Allied army forces in Italy, in 1943 during WWII [47]. Almost simultaneously, it was also described in sick US soldiers stationed in Egypt. Subsequent studies allowed isolation of SFSV in Egypt, India, Iran, Pakistan and Afghanistan [56, 98–100].

Accumulating direct (virus isolation or molecular detection) and indirect (seroprevalence studies) data allowed to list the following countries as areas where SFSV was circulating: Bangladesh, Greece, Cyprus, Iraq, Morocco, Saudi Arabia, Somalia, Ethiopia, Sudan, Tunisia, Turkey, Turkmenia, Tajikistan, Uzbekistan, Azerbaijan, Moldavia, Croatia, Kosovo, France and Portugal [24, 33, 34, 61, 63, 83, 86, 101–103]. Beside the outbreaks described in the Allied and Axis forces during WWII, more recent epidemics were reported in Cyprus, in Turkey and in Ethiopia caused by genetic variants [29–36, 104]. Recent seroprevalence studies provided evidence that SFSV and its genetic variants were still actively circulating in Greece, Cyprus, Portugal and Kosovo [83, 84, 86]. Although *Phlebotomus papatasi, Phlebotomus ariasi* and *P. major* complex were indisputably identified as SFSV vectors, transmission might also be done by phlebotomies belonging to other species [20, 100].

2.1.4 Adria virus

Adria virus was first detected in 2005 from field-collected sandflies in Albania [39]. Genetic data consisting of partial sequence in the polymerase gene showed that Adria virus is much closely related with viruses belonging to the *Salehabad* species than with other phleboviruses belonging to the *Sandfly fever Naples* or to the *Sandfly fever Sicilian* species. In 2009, a 30-month-old patient was admitted to hospital in Greece for fever and seizure during summertime; his blood was tested positive for the presence of phlebovirus RNA, whose sequence was most closely related with Adria virus sequence [23]. Adria virus is the first, and so far the only member of the *Salehabad* species to be associated with human disease. Interestingly, the number of viruses identified in this species has drastically increased during the last decade. Thus efforts should now be deployed to investigate to what extent, Adria virus in particular but also other newly recognized *Salehabad* viruses have a medical impact.

2.1.5 Other phleboviruses

The last decade has been marked by discovery of an unprecedented number of sandfly-borne phleboviruses in old world phlebotomies. Although most of the remains to be classified or listed by the ICTV, they each belong to one of the three species aforementioned: *Sandfly fever Naples, Sandfly fever Sicilian or Salehabad*. Accordingly, they have drastically increased the genetic diversity within each of these species. Since several of these viruses were discovered in sandflies trapped in countries where phleboviruses had never been described before, the geographic range of circulation of the phleboviruses transmitted by sandflies has dramatically expanded.

Sandfly fever Naples species shows an important genetic diversity which has motivated a proposed subdelineation into four groups [42]: subgroup I includes Tehran virus (Iran), Zerdali virus (Turkey) and Sandfly fever Naples virus strain YU 8–76 (Serbia); subgroup II contains the three genotypes of Toscana virus; subgroup III includes Sandfly fever Naples virus and subgroup IV comprises Massilia virus (France), Arrabiata virus (Portugal), Granada virus (Spain) and Punique virus (Tunisia) [11, 18, 37, 42, 46, 47, 105]. Whether viruses belonging to subgroup I and IV can infect humans and may cause disease is currently unknown.

Genetic and phylogenetic analyses show that viruses that can be grouped into the Sandfly fever Sicilian/Corfou virus group or tentative species can be subdivided into two clusters: (i) lineage I contains Sandfly fever Sicilian viruses together with the newly isolated Dashli virus [43] and (ii) lineage II includes Corfou virus together with Toros virus which were isolated from Greece and Turkey, respectively [42, 89].

During the last decade, the *Salehabad virus species* which contained initially only Salehabad and Arbia viruses has greatly increased by addition of newly discovered viruses such as Adana virus, Alcube virus and Medjerda Valley virus, respectively, isolated from sandflies collected in Turkey, Portugal and Tunisia [37–40, 106]. Several other viruses were not isolated but discovered through sequencing a part of their genome such as Adria virus (Albania and Greece), Edirne virus (Turkey) and Olbia virus (France) [23, 39, 107, 108]. To date, Adria virus is the only virus belonging to the *Salehabad species* that was associated with a case of human disease.

Although a large number of these viruses have not been associated with cases of human or veterinarian diseases, it must be remembered that 12 years have passed between the discovery of Toscana virus and the first evidence that it was pathogenic for humans. It is, therefore, crucial to address the public health impacts of these newly described phleboviruses via seroprevalence studies and molecular virological investigations of clinical cases of fever of unknown origin and infections of the central nervous system during summer.

2.2 Sandfly-borne phleboviruses in the new world

2.2.1 Punta Toro virus

Medically speaking, it is the most important phlebovirus in the Americas. Punta Toro virus (PTV) was first identified in the blood of a febrile soldier who participated in military training in the jungle of the Panama Canal Zone, in 1966 [109]. PTV was isolated for the second time in the blood of an entomologist who was doing field collection of insects in the forested area of Darien Province in Panama [108]. Fever, headache, weakness, back, and retro-orbital pain were the common symptoms in both cases with 3–4 days duration. Several Punta Toro virus strains were isolated from sandflies and wild sentinel hamsters in Bayano district of Panama between 1975 and 1976 [109]. To date, PTV has been described only in Central America where several strains of the virus isolated from *Lutzomyia (Nyssomyia) trapidoi* and *L. (Ny.) ylephiletor* [16]. One strain was isolated from the blood of an apparently healthy wild-caught sloth in central Panama [110]. In 1974, a seroprevalence study showed that 5% of the children under the age of 20 and 27–40% of adults in Panama had specific antibodies [111]. In 2009, during the dengue surveillance programme in Panama, dengue virus-negative human samples were found to contain PTV RNA strains. Of the 201 tested sera from febrile patients, 27 (13.4%) were positive for PTV [112].

PTV has been used in several experimental studies [113–115]. Interestingly, when Syrian golden hamsters are inoculated with the Adames strain (PTV-A), they develop a fatal disease; in contrast, hamsters infected with the Baillet strain (PTV-B) do develop a disease but all survive the challenge [113].

2.2.2 Other phleboviruses

A large number of phleboviruses have been isolated from sandflies in Brazil, Panama and Peru [116, 117]. Several viruses have been classified into one the five following groups or species: *Punta Toro, Candiru, Bujaru, Tapara* and *Frijoles species*. However, those which were not classified were included in the tentative species category.

Cocle virus (*Punta Toro species*) was isolated from the serum of a febrile patient in Cocle province, Panama in 2009 [109]. Although it appears that Cocle virus belongs to a species which contains viruses transmitted by sandflies, the absence of entomological data does not allow to conclude about the vector involved in the natural cycle.

Oriximina, Turuna, and Ariquemes viruses (*Candiru species*) were isolated from *Lutzomyia sp.* sandflies in Brazil and Nique virus was isolated from *Lutzomyia panamensis* in Madre de Dios, Peru [116]. Although several viruses belonging to the *Candiru virus species* were identified from febrile patients, there is limited knowledge about the nature of the insect species that transmit these viruses.

3. Other pathogenic sandfly-borne viruses

3.1 *Rhabdoviridae* family

The *Rhabdoviridae* family includes 18 genera and 134 species with negative-sense, single-stranded RNA genomes [118]. In this family, members of the *Vesiculovirus* genus are able to infect at least 28 invertebrates and vertebrates including human [27, 119]. They cause vesicular stomatitis in human and domestic animals and they show a worldwide distribution both in the new and old worlds.

The disease manifests itself into two different forms in the United States; either as sporadic outbreaks with a 10-year intervals in the southwestern states (New Mexico, Arizona, Utah and Colorado) [120]. However, in some other states as Georgia, Alabama, North and South Carolina, the disease occurred yearly with clinical signs in cattle, pig and horses. Since 1970, viral activity has been focal and limited to isolated wildlife populations. [120]. In addition, the virus is considered as endemic in Colombia, Venezuela, Ecuador, Peru and Mexico, where outbreaks occur every year [121, 122].

In the old world, another vesiculovirus, Chandipura virus has recently emerged and caused severe encephalitis in human in different parts of India [6, 123]. The first isolation of Chandipura virus was from two patients with febrile illness in 1965 [6]. In 2003, the virus caused the first outbreak of acute encephalitis in children with high fatality rate (183 deaths out of 329 cases, 55.6%) in Andhra Pradesh, India [124]. The second outbreak has occurred in the eastern state of Gujarat with higher fatality rate in 2004 (>75%) [123]. Recently, an outbreak of acute encephalitis syndrome was recorded in Maharashtra, India with 43.6% fatality rate in children younger than 15-year-old [125].

Chandipura virus has been isolated from field-collected *Phlebotomus spp.* sandflies [7]. The virus was also detected in sandflies belonging to the genus *Sergentomyia* in India [126]. This virus has not only been detected in India but also in Senegal and Nigeria, respectively, from phlebotomine sandflies and hedgehog (*Atelerix spiculus*) [127]. This suggests that Chandipura virus is widely distributed and should be investigated in a more detailed manner.

3.2 Reoviridae family

Changuinola virus was first isolated from *Lutzomyia sp.* sandflies in 1960 in Panama [128]. Since then 12 isolates were described from phlebotomine flies [129]. Another, seven strains were isolated from 80 wild-trapped sloths (*Bradypus variegatus* and *Choloepus hoffmanni)* from Central Panamá [109]. Neutralizing antibody were detected in these two sloth species, despite they were virtually absent from other wild vertebrate species tested. Several strains were associated with prolonged or recrudescent viremias in slots [130]. Besides, one strain of Changuinola virus was identified from a febrile patient [8]. Changuinola virus can replicate in mosquito cell lines (C6/36 [*Aedes albopictus* cells]), *Culicoides sonorensis* KC and African green monkey kidney Vero cells [131].

4. Conclusions

Sandfly-borne viral pathogens are widespread in both old and new worlds particularly in tropical/subtropical areas, and temperate zones including southern Europe, Asia, Africa, Australia and Central and South America [24]. Due to vector sandfly species activity, the sandfly-borne viral diseases peaks during summer which affect both urban, peri-urban and rural population, but mostly the communities with poor living conditions [3, 4] (**Figure 1**, **Table 1**).

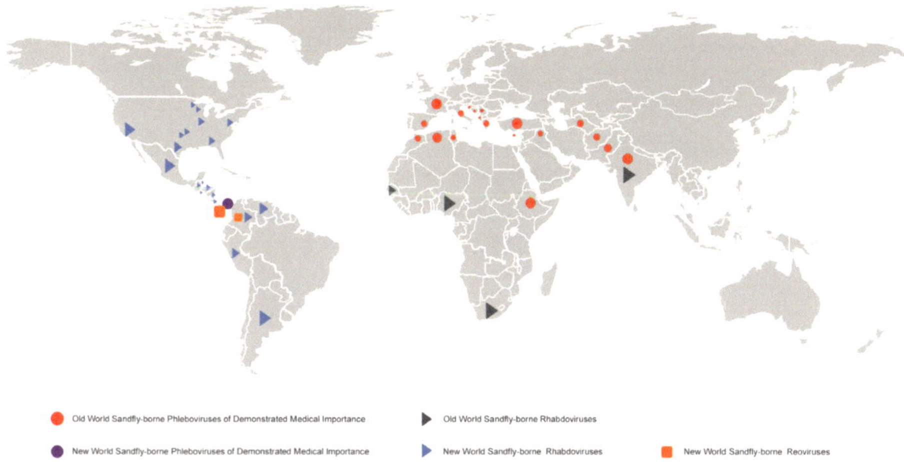

Figure 1.
Schematic overview of the sandfly-brone viruses, according to geographical regions.

Group	Virus	Virus origin	Country
Sandfly-borne phleboviruses of demonstrated medical importance			
Old World Sandfly-borne phleboviruses of demonstrated medical importance			
Sandfly fever Naples Species	Sandfly fever Naples virus Sabin	Blood sample	Italy
	Sandfly fever Naples virus R-3	Human sera	Cyprus
	Sandfly fever Naples virus Namru	*Phlebotomus papatasi*	Egypt
	Sandfly fever Naples virus	Human	Turkmenistan
	Sandfly fever Naples virus	Human	Afghanistan
	Sandfly fever Naples virus	*Phlebotomus longicuspis*	Algeria
	Sandfly fever Naples virus	*Phlebotomus spp.* and humans	India
	Sandfly fever Naples virus YU 8-76	*Phlebotomus perfiliewi*	Serbia
	Toscana virus	*Phlebotomus perniciosus*	Italy
	Toscana virus	Human CSF	Italy
	Toscana virus	*Pipistrellus kuhli* brain	Italy
	Toscana virus	*Phlebotomus spp.*	Italy
	Toscana virus	*Phlebotomus perniciosus*	France
	Toscana virus	*Sergentomyia minuta*	France
	Toscana virus	human CSF	Croatia
	Toscana virus	*Phlebotomus neglectus*	Croatia
	Toscana virus	*Phlebotomus spp.*	Cyprus
	Toscana virus	Human sera, urine	Turkey
	Toscana virus	*Phoenicopterus roseus, Pelecanus onocrotalus, Ciconia nigra*	Turkey
	Toscana virus	*Phlebotomus perniciosus*	Morocco
	Toscana virus	*P. longicuspis, P. sergenti*	Morocco

Group	Virus	Virus origin	Country
	Toscana virus	*Phlebotomus spp.*	Algeria
	Toscana virus	*Phlebotomus spp.*	Tunisia
	Toscana virus	Human CSF	Greece
Sandfly Fever Sicillian Species	Sandfly fever Sicilian virus Sabin	Human sera	Italy
	Sandfly fever Sicilian virus	*Phlebotomus spp.*	Iran
	Sandfly fever Sicilian virus	Human sera	Cyprus
	Sandfly fever Sicilian virus	*Phlebotomus papatasi*	Pakistan
	Sandfly fever Sicilian virus	*Phlebotomus ariasi*	Algeria
	Sandfly fever Sicilian virus	*Phlebotomus papatasi*	Algeria
	Sandfly fever Sicilian virus	Human	Afghanistan
	Sandfly fever Sicilian virus	*Phlebotomus spp.*	India
	Sandfly fever Sicilian virus	Human	Ethiopia
	Sandfly fever Cyprus virus	Human sera	Cyprus
	Sandfly fever Turkey virus	Human sera	Turkey
	Sandfly fever Turkey virus	*Phlebotomus major* complex	Turkey
	Dashli virus	*Phlebotomus spp./ Sergentomyia spp.*	Iran
Salehabad Species	Adria virus	Human blood	Greece
	Adria virus	*Phlebotomus spp.*	Albania
New World Sandfly-borne phleboviruses of demonstrated medical importance			
Punta Toro Species	Punta Toro virus Adames	Human	Panama
	Punta Toro virus Balliet	Human	Panama
	Punta Toro virus	Human	Panama
	Punta Toro virus	Human	Panama
	Punta Toro virus	Sentinel hamster	Panama
	Punta Toro virus	Sentinel hamster	Panama
	Punta Toro virus	*Lutzomyia spp.*	Panama
	Punta Toro virus	Human	Panama
	Punta Toro virus	Human	Panama
	Punta Toro virus	Human	Panama
	Punta Toro virus	Human	Panama
Sandfly-borne Rhabdoviruses			
Vesiculovirus Species	Vesiculovirus	Horse	South Africa
	Vesiculovirus	Bovine	Indiana, USA
	Vesiculovirus	Bovine, equine	New Jersey
	Vesiculovirus	Cattle, horse	Wisconsin, Minnesota, Dakota
	Vesiculovirus	Cattle, horse	Argentine
	Vesiculovirus	Cow, horse, pig	Venezuela
	Vesiculovirus	Horse	Texas, Louisiana
	Vesiculovirus	Horse	Kansas
	Vesiculovirus	Horse	Colorado
	Vesiculovirus	Swine	Colombia

Group	Virus	Virus origin	Country
	Vesiculovirus	Swine	Venezuela
	Vesiculovirus	Swine	Missouri
	Vesiculovirus	Swine	Colorado
	Vesiculovirus	Cattle	California
	Vesiculovirus	Horse	Arizona
	Vesiculovirus	Cattle	Mexico
	Vesiculovirus	Horse	Alabama
	Vesiculovirus	Horse	Mississippi, Georgia, Tennessee, Florida
	Vesiculovirus	Bovine, porcine	Guatemala
	Vesiculovirus	Equine	Belize
	Vesiculovirus	Bovine	Honduras
	Vesiculovirus	Bovine	El Salvador
	Vesiculovirus	Bovine, porcine	Nicaragua
	Vesiculovirus	Bovine	Costa Rica
	Vesiculovirus	Bovine	Peru
	Chandipura virus	Human	India
	Chandipura virus	Sandfly	India
	Chandipura virus	Sandfly	Senegal
	Chandipura virus	Sandfly	Nigeria
Sandfly-borne Reoviruses			
Changuinola virus Species	Changuinola virus	*Lutzomyia sp.*	Panama
	Changuinola virus	Rice rat, armadillo, sloth	Panama
	Changuinola virus	Human	Panama
	Changuinola virus	*Lutzomyia sp.*	Colombia
	Changuinola virus	*Bradypus variegatus, Choloepus hoffmanni*	Panama

Table 1.
Features of the medically important sandfly-borne viruses.

Both molecular characterization and seroepidemiological studies demonstrated broad distribution of sandfly-borne phleboviruses in the old world in the Mediterranean region, in the African continent, in the Indian subcontinent, in the Middle East and in Central Asia. However, the pathogen sandfly-borne phleboviruses were recorded in the limited geographical area (Panama) in the new world with sporadic human cases. This must be due to (i) limited investigations in the new world; (ii) vector competence of phlebovirus in the new world; (iii) small-sized human population and (iv) lack of case report.

Acknowledgements

This work was supported in part by the European Virus Archive goes Global (EVAg) project that has received funding from the European Union's Horizon 2020 research and innovation programme under grant agreement No 653316.
Nazli Ayhan is a Post-Doctoral fellow supported by a IRD grant.

Author details

Nazli Ayhan[1*] and Remi N. Charrel[1,2]

1 Unite des Virus Emergents (Aix-Marseille Univ – IRD 190 – Inserm 1207 – IHU Mediterranee Infection), Marseille, France

2 Emerging Pathogens Institute, University of Florida, Gainesville, Florida, USA

*Address all correspondence to: nazliayhann@gmail.com

References

[1] Killick-Kendrick R. The biology and control of Phlebotomine sand flies. Clinics in Dermatology. 1999;**17**:279-289. DOI: 10.1016/S0738-081X(99)00046-2

[2] Tesh RB. The genus phlebovirus and its vectors. Annual Review of Entomology. 1988;**33**:169-181

[3] Teutsch SM, Churchill RE, editors. Principles and Practice of Public Health Surveillance. USA: Oxford University Press; 2000

[4] Lemon SM, Sparling PF, Hamburg MA, Relmn DA, Choffnes ER, Marck A. Vector-borne diseases: Understanding the environmental, human health, and ecological connections. Workshop summary. In: Vector-Borne Dis Underst Environ Hum Heal Ecol Connect Work Summ. Washington: National Academies Press; 2008

[5] Weaver SC, Reisen WK. Present and future arboviral threats. Antiviral Research. 2010;**85**:328-345

[6] Bhatt PN, Rodrigues FM. Chandipura: A new arbovirus isolated in India from patients with febrile illness. The Indian Journal of Medical Research. 1967;**55**:12

[7] Dhanda V, Rodrigues FM, Ghosh SN. Isolation of Chandipura virus from sandflies in Aurangabad. The Indian Journal of Medical Research. 1970;**58**:179-180

[8] Travassos da Rosa AP, Tesh RB, Pinheiro FP, Travassos da Rosa JP, Peralta PH, Knudson DL. Characterization of the Changuinola serogroup viruses (Reoviridae: Orbivirus). Intervirology. 1984;**21**:38-49. DOI: 10.1159/000149501

[9] Elliott RM, Schmaljohn CS, Collett MS. Bunyaviridae Genome Structure and Gene Expression. Berlin, Heidelberg: Springer; 1991. pp. 91-141. DOI: 10.1007/978-3-642-76018-1_4

[10] Adams MJ, Lefkowitz EJ, King AMQ, et al. Changes to taxonomy and the international code of virus classification and nomenclature ratified by the international committee on taxonomy of viruses. Archives of Virology. 2017;**62**:2505-2538. DOI: 10.1007/s00705-017-3358-5

[11] Zhioua E, Moureau G, Chelbi I, Ninove L, Bichaud L, Derbali M, et al. Punique virus, a novel phlebovirus, related to sandfly fever Naples virus, isolated from sandflies collected in Tunisia. The Journal of General Virology. 2010;**91**:1275-1283. DOI: 10.1099/vir.0.019240-0

[12] Peyrefitte CN, Grandadam M, Bessaud M, Andry PE, Fouque F, Caro V, et al. Diversity of Phlebotomus perniciosus in Provence, Southeastern France: Detection of two putative new Phlebovirus sequences. Vector Borne and Zoonotic Diseases. 2013;**13**(9):630-636. DOI: 10.1089/vbz.2012.1169

[13] Remoli ME, Fortuna C, Marchi A, Bucci P, Argentini C, Bongiorno G, et al. Viral isolates of a novel putative phlebovirus in the Marche region of Italy. The American Journal of Tropical Medicine and Hygiene. 2014;**90**(4):760-763. DOI: 10.4269/ajtmh.13-0457

[14] Alkan C, Alwassouf S, Piorkowski G, Bichaud L, Tezcan S, Dincer E, et al. Isolation, genetic characterization, and seroprevalence of Adana virus, a novel phlebovirus belonging to the salehabad virus complex, in Turkey. Journal of Virology. 2015:03027-03014. DOI: 10.1128/JVI.03027-14

[15] Tesh RB, Lubroth J, Guzman H. Simulation of arbovirus overwintering: Survival of Toscana virus (Bunyaviridae: Phlebovirus) in its natural sand fly vector philebotomus perniciosus. The American Journal of Tropical Medicine and Hygiene. 1992;**47**:574-581. DOI: 10.4269/ajtmh.1992.47.574

[16] Depaquit J, Grandadam M, Fouque F, Andry PE, Peyrefitte C. Arthropod-borne viruses transmitted by Phlebotomine sandflies in Europe: A review. Eurosurveillance. 2010;**15**(10):19507

[17] Alkan C, Bichaud L, De Lamballerie X, Alten B, Gould EA, Charrel RN. Sandfly-borne phleboviruses of Eurasia and Africa: Epidemiology, genetic diversity, geographic range, control measures. Antiviral Research. 2013;**100**(1):54-74. DOI: 10.1016/j.antiviral.2013.07.005

[18] Verani P, Ciufolini MG, Nicoletti L, Balducci M, Sabatinelli G, Coluzzi M, et al. Ecological and epidemiological studies of Toscana virus, an arbovirus isolated from Phlebotomus. Annali dell'Istituto Superiore di Sanità. 1982;**18**:397-399

[19] Coluzzi M, Sabatinelli G, Paci P, Renzi A, Amaducci L, Ciufolini MG, et al. Ecology of viruses isolated from sand flies in Italy and characterization of a new phlebovirus (Arbia virus). The American Journal of Tropical Medicine and Hygiene. 1988;**38**:433-439

[20] Hacioglu S, Dincer E, Isler CT, Karapinar Z, Ataseven VS, Ozkul A, et al. A snapshot avian surveillance reveals west nile virus and evidence of wild birds participating in Toscana cirus circulation. Vector Borne and Zoonotic Diseases. 2017;**17**:698-708. DOI: 10.1089/vbz.2017.2138

[21] Kay MK, Gibney KB, Riedo FX, Kosoy OL, Lanciotti RS, Lambert AJ. Toscana virus infection in American traveler returning from Sicily, 2009. Emerging Infectious Diseases. 2010;**16**:1498-1500. DOI: 10.3201/eid1609.100505

[22] Epelboin L, Hausfater P, Schuffenecker I, Riou B, Zeller H, Bricaire F, et al. Meningoencephalitis due to Toscana virus in a French traveler returning from Central Italy. Journal of Travel Medicine. 2008;**15**:361-363. DOI: 10.1111/j.1708-8305.2008.00221.x

[23] Anagnostou V, Pardalos G, Athanasiou-Metaxa M, Papa A. Novel phlebovirus in febrile child, Greece. Emerging Infectious Diseases. 2011;**17**:940. DOI: 10.3201/eid1705.101958

[24] Tesh RB, Saidi S, Gajdamovic SJ, Rodhain F, Vesenjak-Hirjan J. Serological studies on the epidemiology of sandfly fever in the Old World. Bulletin of the World Health Organization. 1976;**54**:663-674

[25] Alivisatos GP. The Outbreak of Three-Day Fever at Athens in 1935. Bulletin de l'Office International d'Hygiene Publique. 1936;**28**(11):2146-2166.

[26] Tesh RB, Papaevangelou G. Effect of insecticide spraying for malaria control on the incidence of sandfly fever in Athens, Greece. The American Journal of Tropical Medicine and Hygiene. 1977;**26**:163-166. DOI: 10.4269/ajtmh.1977.26.163

[27] Maroli M, Feliciangeli MD, Bichaud L, Charrel RN, Gradoni L. Phlebotomine sandflies and the spreading of leishmaniases and other diseases of public health concern. Medical and Veterinary Entomology. 2013;**27**(2):123-147. DOI: 10.1111/j.1365-2915.2012.01034.x

[28] Karakašević BO. Prvoj epidemiji papatačijeve groznice na teritoriji NR Srbije. Vojnosanitetski Pregled. 1947;**4**:224-228

[29] Vesenjak-Hirjan J, Punda-Polić V, Dobe M. Geographical distribution of arboviruses in Yugoslavia. Journal of Hygiene, Epidemiology, Microbiology, and Immunology. 1991;**35**:129-140

[30] Hukić M, Numanović F, Šiširak M, Moro A, Dervović E, Jakovac S, et al. Surveillance of wildlife zoonotic diseases in the Balkans region. Medicinski Glasnik. 2010;**7**(2)

[31] Hukić M, Bešić IS. Sandfly-Pappataci fever in Bosnia and Herzegovina: The new-old disease. Bosnian Journal of Basic Medical Sciences. 2009;**9**(1):39

[32] Simic C. O posleratnoj pojavi papatacˇijeve groznice u Srbiji i Banatu. Glas Srpske akademije nauka CCIV. Odjeljenje Medicinskih Nauka. 1951;**4**:143-152

[33] Ahmed A, Abera NA, Cao S, Omballa V, Wang D, Montgomery JM, et al. An outbreak of acute febrile illness caused by sandfly fever Sicilian virus in the Afar region of Ethiopia, 2011. The American Journal of Tropical Medicine and Hygiene. 2014;**91**:1250-1253. DOI: 10.4269/ajtmh.14-0299

[34] Papa A, Konstantinou G, Pavlidou V, Antoniadis A. Sandfly fever virus outbreak in Cyprus. Clinical Microbiology and Infection. 2006;**12**:192-194. DOI: 10.1111/j.1469-0691.2005.01330.x

[35] Ellis SB, Appenzeller G, Lee H, Mullen K, Swenness R, Pimentel G, et al. Outbreak of sandFly fever in Central Iraq, September 2007. Military Medicine. 2008;**173**:949-953. DOI: 10.7205/MILMED.173.10.949

[36] Guler S, Guler E, Caglayik DY, Kokoglu OF, Ucmak H, Bayrakdar F, et al. A sandfly fever virus outbreak in the East Mediterranean region of Turkey. International Journal of Infectious Diseases. 2012;**16**:e244-e246. DOI: 10.1016/j.ijid.2011.12.001

[37] Amaro F, Hanke D, Zé-Zé L, Alves MJ, Becker SC, Höper D. Genetic characterization of Arrabida virus, a novel phlebovirus isolated in South Portugal. Virus Research. 2016;**214**:19-25. DOI: 10.1016/J.VIRUSRES.2016.01.004

[38] Amaro F, Zé-Zé L, Alves MJ, Alves MJ, Börstler J, Clos J, et al. Co-circulation of a novel phlebovirus and Massilia virus in sandflies, Portugal. Virology Journal. 2011;**17**(4):585-587. DOI: 10.1186/s12985-015-0407-0

[39] Papa A, Velo E, Bino S. A novel phlebovirus in Albanian sandflies. Clinical Microbiology and Infection. 2011;**17**:585-587

[40] Ayhan N, Velo E, De Lamballerie X, Kota M, Kadriaj P, Ozbel Y, et al. Detection of Leishmania infantum and a novel Phlebovirus (Balkan virus) from sand flies in Albania. Vector Borne and Zoonotic Diseases. 2016;**16**(12):802-806. DOI: 10.1089/vbz.2016.2002

[41] Ayhan N, Alten B, Ivovic V, Dvořák V, Martinkovic F, Omeragic J, et al. Direct evidence for an expanded circulation area of the recently identified Balkan virus (Sandfly fever Naples virus species) in several countries of the Balkan archipelago. Parasites & Vectors. 2017;**10**(1). DOI: 10.1186/s13071-017-2334-y

[42] Alkan C, Erisoz Kasap O, Alten B, De Lamballerie X, Charrel RN. Sandfly-borne phlebovirus isolations from Turkey: New insight into the sandfly fever sicilian and sandfly fever Naples species. PLoS Neglected Tropical Diseases. 2016;**10**:e0004519. DOI: 10.1371/journal.pntd.0004519

[43] Alkan C, Moin Vaziri V, Ayhan N, Badakhshan M, Bichaud L, Rahbarian N, et al. Isolation and sequencing of Dashli virus, a novel Sicilian-like virus in sandflies from Iran; genetic and phylogenetic evidence for the

creation of one novel species within the Phlebovirus genus in the Bunyaviridae family. PLoS Neglected Tropical Diseases. 2017;**11**(12). DOI: 10.1371/journal.pntd.0005978

[44] Aspöck H, Gerersdorfer T, Formayer H, Walochnik J. Sandflies and sandfly-borne infections of humans in Central Europe in the light of climate change. Wiener Klinische Wochenschrift. 2008;**120**(4):24-29. DOI: 10.1007/s00508-008-1072-8

[45] Charrel RN, Gallian P, Navarro-Marí JM, Nicoletti L, Papa A, Sánchez-Seco MP, et al. Emergence of Toscana virus in Europe. Emerging Infectious Diseases. 2005;**11**(11):1657. DOI: 10.3201/eid1111.050869

[46] Charrel RN, Moureau G, Temmam S, Izri A, Marty P, Parola P, et al. Massilia virus, a novel Phlebovirus (Bunyaviridae) isolated from sandflies in the Mediterranean. Vector Borne and Zoonotic Diseases. 2009;**9**(5):519-530. DOI: 10.1089/vbz.2008.0131

[47] Sabin AB. Experimental studies on phlebotomus (pappataci, sandfly) fever during world war II. Archiv für die Gesamte Virusforschung. 1951;**4**(4):367-410. DOI: 10.1007/BF01241161

[48] Doerr R, Franz KTS. Das Papatatsi Fieber. Franz Deuticke, Leipzig- Wien; 1909

[49] Taussig S. Die Hundskrankheit, endemischer Magenkatarrh in der Herzegowina. Wiener klinische Wochenschrift. 1905;**50**:164

[50] Livschitz J. Studies on Pappataci fever. Medical Parasitology and Parasitic Diseases (Moscow). 1937;**6**:938-943

[51] Shortt HE, Poole LT, Stephens ED. Sandfly fever on the Indian frontier. A preliminary note on some laboratory investigations. The Indian Journal of Medical Research. 1934;**21**:775-788

[52] Anderson WME. Clinical observations on sandfly fever in the Peshawar district. Journal of the Royal Army Medical Corps. 1941;77:225-239

[53] Maroli M, Feliciangeli MD, Bichaud L, Charrel RN, Gradoni L. Phlebotomine sandflies and the spreading of leishmaniases and other diseases of public health concern. Medical and Veterinary Entomology. 2013;**27**:123-147. DOI: 10.1111/j.1365-2915.2012.01034.x

[54] American Society of Tropical Medicine and Hygiene. AB. The American Journal of Tropical Medicine and Hygiene. Allen Press; 1955

[55] Československá Akademie Věd SY, Kurakhmedova SA, Melnikova EE. Acta Virologica. Academia, Pub. House of the Czechoslovak Academy of Sciences; 1974

[56] Goverdhan MK, Dhanda V, Modi GB, Bhatt PN, Bhagwat RB, Dandawate CN, et al. Isolation of phlebotomus (sandfly) fever virus from sandflies and humans during the same season in Aurangabad District, Maharashtra state, India. The Indian Journal of Medical Research. 1976;**64**:57-63

[57] Gaidamovich SY, Khutoretskaya NV, Asyamov YV, Tsyupa VI, Melnikova EE. Sandfly fever in Central Asia and Afghanistan. In: Hemorrhagic Fever with Renal Syndrome, Tick- and Mosquito-Borne Viruses. Vienna: Springer Vienna; 1990. pp. 287-293. DOI: 10.1007/978-3-7091-9091-3_32

[58] Ennis WH, Peters CJ, Feinsod FM, et al. Sand fly fever-Naples infection in Egypt. The American Journal of Tropical Medicine and Hygiene. 1987;**37**:193-196. DOI: 10.4269/ajtmh.1987.37.193

[59] Schmidt JR, Schmidt ML, Said MI, Soliman AK, Farrag IH, El Said S, et al. Phlebotomus fever in Egypt. The American Journal of Tropical Medicine and Hygiene. 1971;**20**:483-490. DOI: 10.4269/ajtmh.1971.20.483

[60] Darwish MA, Feinsod FM, Scott RM, Ksiazek TG, Botros BAM, Farrag IH, et al. Arboviral causes of non-specific fever and myalgia in a fever hospital patient population in Cairo, Egypt. Transactions of the Royal Society of Tropical Medicine and Hygiene. 1987;**81**:1001-1003

[61] Eitrem R, Vene S, Niklasson B. Incidence of sand fly fever among Swedish United Nations soldiers on Cyprus during 1985. The American Journal of Tropical Medicine and Hygiene. 1990;**43**:207-211. DOI: 10.1016/0035-9203(87)90378-6

[62] Gligić A, Mišcević Z, Tesh RB, Travassos da Rosa AZV. First isolations of Naples sandfly fever virus in Yugoslavia. Mikrobiologija. 1982;**19**:167-175

[63] Gaidamovich SI, Obukhova VR, Sveshnikova NA, Cherednichenko IN, Kostiukov MA. Natural foci of viruses borne by Phlebotomus papatasi in the USSR according to a serologic study of the population. Voprosy Virusologii. 1978:556-560

[64] Ehrnst A, Peters CJ, Niklasson B, Svedmyr A, Holmgren B. Neurovirulent Toscana virus (a sandfly fever virus) in Swedish man after visit to Portugal. Lancet (London, England). 1985;**1**:1212-1213

[65] Calisher CH, Weinberg AN, Muth DJ, Lazuick JS. Toscana virus infection in United States citizen returning from Italy. Lancet (London, England). 1987;**1**:165-166

[66] Schwarz TF, Gilch S, Jäger G. Travel-related Toscana virus infection. Lancet (London, England). 1993;**342**:803-804

[67] Dobler G, Treib J, Haass A, Frösner G, Woesner R, Schimrigk K. Toscana virus infection in German travellers returning from the Mediterranean. Infection. 1997;**25**(5):325-325

[68] Eitrem R, Niklasson B, Weiland O. Sandfly fever among Swedish tourists. Scandinavian Journal of Infectious Diseases. 1991;**23**:451-457

[69] Veater J, Mehedi F, Cheung CK, Nabarro L, Osborne J, Wong N, et al. Toscana virus meningo-encephalitis: An important differential diagnosis for elderly travellers returning from Mediterranean countries. BMC Geriatrics. 2017;**17**:193. DOI: 10.1186/s12877-017-0593-2

[70] Arden KE, Heney C, Shaban B, Nimmo GR, Nissen MD, Sloots TP, et al. Detection of Toscana virus from an adult traveler returning to Australia with encephalitis. Journal of Medical Virology. 2017;**89**:1861-1864. DOI: 10.1002/jmv.24839

[71] Renzi A, Caciolli S, Nicoletti L, Bartolozzi D, Balducci M, Traini E, et al. Central nervous system involvement during infection by Phlebovirus Toscana of residents in natural foci in Central Italy (1977-1988). The American Journal of Tropical Medicine and Hygiene. 1991;**45**:429-434. DOI: 10.4269/ajtmh.1991.45.429

[72] Papa A, Paraforou T, Papakonstantinou I, Pagdatoglou K, Kontana A, Koukoubani T. Severe encephalitis caused by Toscana virus, Greece. Emerging Infectious Diseases. 2014;**20**:1417-1419. DOI: 10.3201/eid2008.140248

[73] Eitrem R, Stylianou M, Niklasson B. High prevalence rates of antibody to three sandfly fever viruses (Sicilian, Naples and Toscana) among

Cypriots. Epidemiology and Infection. 1991;**107**:685-691. DOI: 10.1017/S0950268800049384

[74] Punda-Polić V, Mohar B, Duh D, Bradarić N, Korva M, Fajs L, et al. Evidence of an autochthonous Toscana virus strain in Croatia. Journal of Clinical Virology. 2012;**55**:4-7. DOI: 10.1016/j.jcv.2012.06.006

[75] Kuşcu F, Menemenlioğlu D, Oztürk DB, Korukluoğlu G, Uyar Y. Acute Toscana virus infection in an anti-HIV positive patient. Mikrobiyoloji Bülteni. 2014;**48**:168-173

[76] Ocal M, Orsten S, Inkaya AC, Yetim E, Acar NP, Alp S, et al. Ongoing activity of Toscana virus genotype a and West Nile virus lineage 1 strains in Turkey: A clinical and field survey. Zoonoses and Public Health. 2014;**61**:480-491. DOI: 10.1111/zph.12096

[77] Santos L, Simões J, Costa R, Martins S, Lecour H. Toscana virus meningitis in Portugal, 2002-2005. Euro Surveillance. 2007;**2**:E3-E4

[78] Peyrefitte CN, Devetakov I, Pastorino B, et al. Toscana virus and acute meningitis, France. Emerging Infectious Diseases. 2005;**11**:778-780. DOI: 10.3201/EID1105.041122

[79] Karunaratne K, Nicholas D. Toscana virus meningitis following a holiday in Elba, Italy. British Journal of Hospital Medicine (London, England: 2005). 2018;**79**(5):292. DOI: 10.12968/hmed.2018.79.5.292

[80] Gabriel M, Resch C, Günther S, Schmidt-Chanasit J. Toscana virus infection imported from Elba into Switzerland. Emerging Infectious Diseases. 2010;**16**(6):1034. DOI: 10.3201/eid1606.091763

[81] Kay MK, Gibney KB, Riedo FX, Kosoy OL, Lanciotti RS, Lambert AJ. Toscana virus infection in American traveler returning from Sicily, 2009. Emerging Infectious Diseases. 2010;**16**(9):1498. DOI: 10.3201/eid1609.100505

[82] Dupouey J, Bichaud L, Ninove L, Zandotti C, Thirion-Perrier L, De Lamballerie X, et al. Toscana virus infections: A case series from France. The Journal of Infection. 2014;**68**(3):290-295. DOI: 10.1016/j.jinf.2013.11.006

[83] Alwassouf S, Maia C, Ayhan N, Coimbra M, Cristovao JM, Richet H, et al. Neutralization-based seroprevalence of Toscana virus and sandfly fever sicilian virus in dogs and cats from Portugal. The Journal of General Virology. 2016;**97**(11):2816-2823. DOI: 10.1099/jgv.0.000592

[84] Alwassouf S, Christodoulou V, Bichaud L, et al. Seroprevalence of sandfly-borne Phleboviruses belonging to three serocomplexes (sandfly fever Naples, sandfly fever sicilian and salehabad) in dogs f rom Greece and Cyprus using neutralization test. PLoS Neglected Tropical Diseases. 2016;**10**:e0005063. DOI: 10.1371/journal.pntd.0005063

[85] Tahir D, Alwassouf S, Loudahi A, Davoust B, Charrel RN. Seroprevalence of Toscana virus in dogs from Kabylia (Algeria). Clinical Microbiology and Infection. 2016;**22**(3):e16-e17. DOI: 10.1016/j.cmi.2015.10.029

[86] Ayhan N, Sherifi K, Taraku A, Bërxholi K, Charrel RN. High rates of neutralizing antibodies to Toscana and sandfly fever Sicilian viruses in livestock, Kosovo. Emerging Infectious Diseases. 2017;**23**:989-992. DOI: 10.3201/eid2306.161929

[87] Alkan C, Allal-Ikhlef AB, Alwassouf S, Baklouti A, Piorkowski G, de Lamballerie X, et al. Virus isolation, genetic characterization

and seroprevalence of Toscana virus in Algeria. Clinical Microbiology and Infection. 2015;**21**:1040.e1-1040.e9. DOI: 10.1016/j.cmi.2015.07.012

[88] Pierro A, Ficarelli S, Ayhan N, Morini S, Raumer L, Bartoletti M, et al. Characterization of antibody response in neuroinvasive infection caused by Toscana virus. Clinical Microbiology and Infection. 2017;**23**(11):868-873. DOI: 10.1016/j.cmi.2017.03.017

[89] Rodhain F, Madulo-Leblond G, Hannoun C, Tesh RB. Le virus Corfou: Un nouveau phlebovirus isolé de phlébotomes en Grèce. Annales de l'Institut Pasteur Virologie. 1985;**136**:161-166. DOI: 10.1016/S0769-2617(85)80042-3

[90] Ergünay K, Litzba N, Lo MM, Aydoğan S, Saygan MB, Us D, et al. Performance of various commercial assays for the detection of Toscana virus antibodies. Vector Borne and Zoonotic Diseases. 2011;**11**(6):781-787. DOI: 10.1089/vbz.2010.0224

[91] Charrel RN, Izri A, Temmam S, Delaunay P, Toga I, Dumon H, et al. Cocirculation of 2 genotypes of Toscana virus, southeastern France. Emerging Infectious Diseases. 2007;**13**:465. DOI: 10.3201/eid1303.061086

[92] Charrel RN, Izri A, Temmam S, De Lamballerie X, Parola P. Toscana virus RNA in Sergentomyia minuta files. Emerging Infectious Diseases. 2006;**12**. DOI: 1299. DOI:10.3201/eid1208.060345

[93] Ayhan N, Alten B, Ivovic V, Martinkovic F, Kasap OE, Ozbel Y, et al. Cocirculation of two lineages of Toscana virus in Croatia. Frontiers in Public Health. 2017;**5**:336. DOI: 10.3389/fpubh.2017.00336

[94] Es-sette N, Ajaoud M, Anga L, Mellouki F, Lemrani M. Toscana virus isolated from sandflies, Morocco. Parasites & Vectors. 2015;**8**:205. DOI: 10.1186/s13071-015-0826-1

[95] Bichaud L, Dachraoui K, Piorkowski G, Chelbi I, Moureau G, Cherni S, et al. Toscana virus isolated from sandflies, Tunisia. Emerging Infectious Diseases. 2013;**19**:322. DOI: 10.3201/EID1902.121463

[96] Bichaud L, Izri A, de Lamballerie X, Moureau G, Charrel RN. First detection of Toscana virus in Corsica, France. Clinical Microbiology and Infection. 2014;**20**(2):101-104. DOI: 10.1111/1469-0691.12347

[97] Dincer E, Ozkul A, Gargari S, Ergunay K. Potential animal reservoirs of Toscana virus and coinfections with Leishmania infantum in Turkey. The American Journal of Tropical Medicine and Hygiene. 2015;**92**:690-697. DOI: 10.4269/ajtmh.14-0322

[98] Gaĭdamovich SI, Khutoretskaia NV, Aziamov IV, Tsiupa VI, Melnikova EE. Virological study of cases of sandfly fever in Afghanistan. Voprosy Virusologii. 1990;**35**:45-47

[99] Javadian E, Saidi S, Tesh R, Nadim A. Studies on the epidemiology of Sandfly fever in Iran. The American Journal of Tropical Medicine and Hygiene. 1977;**26**:282-287. DOI: 10.4269/ajtmh.1977.26.282

[100] George JE. Isolation of phlebotomus fever virus from Phlebotomus Papatasi and determination of the host ranges of sandflies (Diptera: Psychodidae) in west Pakistan1. Journal of Medical Entomology. 1970;**7**:670-676. DOI: 10.1093/jmedent/7.6.670

[101] Carhan A, Uyar Y, Ozkaya E, Ertek M, Dobler G, Dilcher M, et al. Characterization of a sandfly fever Sicilian virus isolated during a sandfly fever epidemic in Turkey. Journal of

Clinical Virology. 2010;**48**:264-269. DOI: 10.1016/j.jcv.2010.05.011

[102] Niklasson B, Eitrem R. Sandfly fever among Swedish UN troops in Cyprus. The Lancet. 1985;**325**(8439):1212

[103] Filipe AR. Serological survey for antibodies to arboviruses in the human population of Portugal. Transactions of the Royal Society of Tropical Medicine and Hygiene. 1974;**68**:311-314. DOI: 10.1016/0035-9203(74)90039-X

[104] Ahmed A, Abera NA, Cao S, Omballa V, Wang D, Montgomery JM, et al. An outbreak of acute febrile illness caused by Sandfly fever Sicilian virus in the Afar region of Ethiopia, 2011. The American Journal of Tropical Medicine and Hygiene. 2014;**91**:1250-1253. DOI: 10.4269/ajtmh.14-0299

[105] Collao X, Palacios G, De Ory F, Sanbonmatsu S, Pérez-Ruiz M, Navarro JM, et al. Granada virus: A natural phlebovirus reassortant of the sandfly fever Naples serocomplex with low seroprevalence in humans. The American Journal of Tropical Medicine and Hygiene. 2010;**83**(4):760-765. DOI: 10.4269/ajtmh.2010.09-0697

[106] Bichaud L, Dachraoui K, Alwassouf S, Alkan C, Mensi M, raldine Piorkowski G, et al. Isolation, full genomic characterization and neutralization-based human seroprevalence of Medjerda Valley virus, a novel sandfly-borne phlebovirus belonging to the Salehabad virus complex in northern Tunisia. The Journal of General Virology. 2016;**97**(3):602-610. DOI: 10.1099/jgv.0.000389

[107] Ergunay K, Kasap OE, Orsten S, Oter K, Gunay F, Yoldar AZA, et al. Phlebovirus and Leishmania detection in sandflies from eastern Thrace and northern Cyprus. Parasites & Vectors. 2014;**7**:575. DOI: 10.1186/s13071-014-0575-6

[108] Peyrefitte CN, Grandadam M, Bessaud M, Andry PE, Fouque F, Caro V, et al. Diversity of *Phlebotomus perniciosus* in Provence, Southeastern France: Detection of two putative new phlebovirus sequences. Vector Borne and Zoonotic Diseases. 2013;**13**:630-636. DOI: 10.1089/vbz.2012.1169

[109] Palacios G, Wiley MR, A Travassos da Rosa AP, Guzman H, Quiroz E, Savji N, et al. Characterization of the Punta Toro species complex (genus Phlebovirus, family Bunyaviridae). The Journal of General Virology. 2015;**96**(8):2079-2085. DOI: 10.1099/vir.0.000170

[110] Montgomery GG, Seymour C, Peralta PH. Viruses isolated from Panamanian sloths. The American Journal of Tropical Medicine and Hygiene. 1983;**32**. DOI: 1435-1444. DOI: 10.4269/ajtmh.1983.32.1435

[111] Peralta PH, Tesh RB, Johnson KM, Chaniotis BN. Ecology of viruses isolated from Panamanian phlebotomine sandflies. The American Journal of Tropical Medicine and Hygiene. 1974;**23**:258-269. DOI: 10.4269/ajtmh.1974.23.258

[112] Gundacker ND, Carrera J-P, Castillo M, Díaz Y, Valenzuela J, Tamhane A, et al. Clinical manifestations of Punta Toro virus species complex infections, Panama, 2009. Emerging Infectious Diseases. 2017;**23**:872-874

[113] Anderson GW, Slayter MV, Hall W, Peters CJ. Pathogenesis of a phleboviral infection (Punta Toro virus) in golden Syrian hamsters. Archives of Virology. 1990;**114**:203-212. DOI: 10.1007/BF01310749

[114] Perrone LA, Narayanan K, Worthy M, Peters CJ. The S segment of Punta Toro virus (Bunyaviridae, Phlebovirus)

is a major determinant of lethality in the Syrian hamster and codes for a type I interferon antagonist. Journal of Virology. 2007;**81**:884-892. DOI: 10.1128/JVI.01074-06

[115] Ashley SL, Ameres SM, Gerrard SR, Foreman O, Eaton KA, Weinberg JB, et al. Host genetic variation in susceptibility to Punta Toro virus. Virus Research. 2011;**157**:71-75. DOI: 10.1016/j.virusres.2011.02.008

[116] Palacios G, Tesh R, Travassos Da Rosa A, Savji N, Sze W, Jain K, et al. Characterization of the Candiru antigenic complex (Bunyaviridae: Phlebovirus), a highly diverse and Reassorting Group of Viruses Affecting Humans in tropical America. Journal of Virology. 2011;**85**:3811-3820. DOI: 10.1128/JVI.02275-10

[117] Nunes-Neto JP, de SWM, Acrani GO, Romeiro MF, Fumagalli M, Vieira LC, et al. Characterization of the Bujaru, frijoles and Tapara antigenic complexes into the sandfly fever group and two unclassified phleboviruses from Brazil. The Journal of General Virology. 2017;**98**:585-594. DOI: 10.1099/jgv.0.000724

[118] Walker PJ, Blasdell KR, Calisher CH, Dietzgen RG, Kondo H, Kurath G, et al. ICTV virus taxonomy profile: Rhabdoviridae. The Journal of General Virology. 2018;**99**:447-448. DOI: 10.1099/jgv.0.001020

[119] Wunner WH, Peters D. Rhabdoviridae. In: classification and nomenclature of viruses. 5th Report nternational Committee on Taxonomy of Viruses. 1991;250-262

[120] Rodríguez LL. Emergence and re-emergence of vesicular stomatitis in the United States. Virus Research. 2002;**85**:211-219. DOI: 10.1016/S0168-1702(02)00026-6

[121] Hanson RP, Estupiñan J, Castañeda J. Vesicular stomatitis in the Americas. Bulletin - Office International des Épizooties. 1968;**70**:37-47

[122] Vanleeuwen JA, Waltner-Toews D, Rodriguez LL. Cow, farm, and ecologic risk factors of clinical vesicular stomatitis on Costa Rican dairy farms. The American Journal of Tropical Medicine and Hygiene. 1995;**53**:342-350. DOI: 10.4269/ajtmh.1995.53.342

[123] Chadha MS, Arankalle VA, Jadi RS, et al. An outbreak of Chandipura virus encephalitis in the eastern districts of Gujarat state, India. The American Journal of Tropical Medicine and Hygiene. 2005;**73**:566-570. DOI: 10.4269/ajtmh.2005.73.566

[124] Rao B, Basu A, Wairagkar NS, Arankalle VA, Thakare JP, Jadi RS, et al. A large outbreak of acute encephalitis with high fatality rate in children in Andhra Pradesh, India, in 2003, associated with Chandipura virus. Lancet. 2004;**364**:869-874. DOI: 10.1016/S0140-6736(04)16982-1

[125] Gurav YK, Tandale BV, Jadi RS, Gunjikar RS, Tikute SS, Jamgaonkar AV, et al. Chandipura virus encephalitis outbreak among children in Nagpur division, Maharashtra, 2007. The Indian Journal of Medical Research. 2010;**132**:395

[126] Geevarghese G, Arankalle VA, Jadi R, Kanojia PC, Joshi MV, Mishra AC. Detection of Chandipura virus from sand flies in the genus Sergentomyia (Diptera: Phlebotomidae) at Karimnagar District, Andhra Pradesh, India. Journal of Medical Entomology. 2005;**42**:495-496. DOI: 10.1093/jmedent/42.3.495

[127] Fontenille D, Ba Y, Digoutte JP, Zeller HG, Mondo M, Traore-Lamizana M, et al. First isolations of arboviruses from Phlebotomine sand flies in West Africa. The American Journal of Tropical Medicine and Hygiene.

1994;**50**:570-574. DOI: 10.4269/ajtmh.1994.50.570

[128] Marriott AC. Complete genome sequences of Chandipura and Isfahan vesiculoviruses. Archives of Virology. 2005;**150**:671-680. DOI: 10.1007/s00705-004-0452-2

[129] Mohd Jaafar F, Belhouchet M, Belaganahalli M, Tesh RB, Mertens PPC, Attoui H. Full-genome characterisation of Orungo, Lebombo and Changuinola viruses provides evidence for Co-evolution of Orbiviruses with their arthropod vectors. PLoS One. 2014;**9**:e86392. DOI: 10.1371/journal.pone.0086392

[130] Longfellow D, Shelokov A, Vogel JE, Peralta PH. Isolation and characterization of arboviruses from Almirante, Republic of Panama. The American Journal of Tropical Medicine and Hygiene. 1966;**15**:369-378. DOI: 10.4269/ajtmh.1966.15.3

[131] Karabatsos N. Supplement to international catalogue of arboviruses including certain other viruses of vertebrates. The American Journal of Tropical Medicine and Hygiene. 1978;**27**:372-440

Chapter 5

An Overview of Leishmaniasis: Historic to Future Perspectives

Mümtaz Güran

Abstract

Human leishmaniasis is a major public health problem with a wide clinical spectrum. Despite there is an epidemiological diversity of the disease, cases mostly occur in the developing countries around the subtropical region, and the incidence is significantly rising. The disease is usually classified into three groups: cutaneous leishmaniasis, mucosal leishmaniasis, and visceral leishmaniasis. But to ensure their survival in different conditions, *Leishmania* spp. have developed many adaptation mechanisms and can be seen in different clinical forms as well. Herein, an overview of the characteristics of the disease and the parasite, interactions with the host, clinical aspects, and latest developments in the diagnosis and treatment is presented.

Keywords: leishmaniasis, kala-azar, vector borne diseases

1. Introduction

Human leishmaniasis is a sandfly-mediated parasitic disease that can lead to severe conditions in individuals especially with underdeveloped immune system. It usually affects people living in developing tropical countries and has high mortality rates [1]. Transmission of the parasite starts with an infected sandfly bite. After getting bit by a female sandfly vector carrying the promastigote form of the *Leishmania* protozoan, the promastigotes transform into amastigote form in mammalian hosts [2]. Once amastigotes enter the cells, immune system starts reacting to it. Phagocytes absorb the parasite, and destructive mechanism is initiated in order to kill the parasite. However, parasite has different ways of preventing or lowering the activity of immune system, and three distinct forms of leishmaniasis can be observed as a result which are cutaneous leishmaniasis (CL), visceral leishmaniasis (VL), and mucocutaneous leishmaniasis (ML). CL usually occurs around the uncovered sites such as face, neck, and extremities which are susceptible to sandfly bite and often can result in the formation of ulcers or nodules around exposed areas. In certain conditions, macrophages infected by the parasites at the initial bite site spread among the reticuloendothelial system causing VL. Abnormal growth of internal organs such as the spleen and liver is common in VL, and it can cause death if necessary treatment methods are not applied. Another form of leishmaniasis is the ML in which parasites enter the mucocutaneous tissue, and its effects are usually seen around the oral and upper respiratory tract [3].

Leishmaniasis is considered to be an endemic disease effecting more than 98 countries with a global prevalence of 12 million people. Among different types of disease, CL makes up great percentage of the total amount of cases compared to other two. East Africa, Brazil, and Indian subcontinent are hot spots for VL cases, whereas

IntechOpen

CL cases are high in the Middle East, Mediterranean region, Central Asia, and Latin American countries [4]. In European countries where leishmaniasis is not endemic, people traveling to endemic regions for various reasons such as military duty, tourism work, and vacation are the major cause of leishmaniasis occurrence [5].

There are more than 20 *Leishmania* species responsible from leishmaniasis [3]. In general, *Leishmania* major causes CL, *Leishmania donovani* causes VL, and *Leishmania infantum* results in both CL and VL [3]. These species can be further classified into subgenera depending on anatomical varieties of infection sites. Old World sandfly species are common in desert and semidry areas, whereas New World sandfly species transmit the disease to human near forest habitation [6]. *Leishmania* parasite has promastigote form in sandfly and amastigote form in mammalians. It can be transmitted by the vectors from an animal carrying this parasite or humans affected by VL. Amastigotes develop within the phagocytes and spread to other macrophages as a result of cell lysis. Once a sandfly bites an infected host, amastigotes then transform into promastigote form inside the sandfly restarting the transmission process for the next host that will be infected.

Leishmaniasis is ranked second in mortality right after malaria and ranked fourth in terms of morbidity among other communicable diseases [2]. HIV outbreak in the 1990s resulting in HIV/VL coinfection and general global warming of the world increasing the possible habitat for the sandfly led to doubling the amount of cases from 1987 to 2014 despite developing medical technologies [6]. It is estimated that each year around 400,000 people are having VL with a mortality rate of 10% going up to 20% in some areas [2, 3]. The Mediterranean region, Western Asia, and the Americas make up the 90% of 1 million CL cases, whereas ML is represented by 35,000 cases in these regions [3]. Among the other common forms of the disease, CL has the highest amount of cases reported each year. On the other hand, VL is the most fatal one where death usually occurs 2 years after the first transmission.

There are 98 countries and territories with *Leishmania* cases recorded each year [7]. It affects around 12 million people worldwide, and 1.5–2 million new cases are reported each year. Being an ignored tropical disease, leishmaniasis has the highest prevalence in poor countries such as India, Brazil, Ethiopia, and Afghanistan. Notably, there has been an increase in the CL case reports for Syria in the Middle East, Algeria in the Mediterranean, and India [6]. Poor housing, insufficient sanitary conditions, poor waste management, poverty, malnutrition, and change in climate conditions such as temperature, rainfall, and humidity are common features of these countries. Children living in these countries are considered the main reason of parasite transmission as they are the most vulnerable population group to sandfly bite.

Among species, *L. major* shows the biggest geographical distribution in the Middle East region compared to *Leishmania tropica* and *Leishmania infantum* [8]. *L. infantum* caused zoonotic and *L. tropica* caused anthroponotic transmissions to occur. Domestic dogs, rodents, and wild animals in endemic regions hold epidemiological importance as they take part in transmission of the parasite by serving as reservoirs.

Parasites can only reach infective stages in certain species of sandfly which as a result limits its transmission [9]. In addition, parasite-vector contact is rare for great majority of the sandfly species [10]. Epidemiological concerns about the leishmaniasis have increased greatly in the last 30 years. HIV/*Leishmania* coinfection, sandflies becoming more apparent in areas that they were less present such as the United States and Canada, and great risk of *Leishmania* gaining resistance to drugs over time make it a high-risk factor globally [11]. Another major concern for leishmaniasis is the increased resistance gain by parasite to current treatment methods which makes it even more dangerous considering there is an ongoing effort to develop a human vaccine against the disease [12].

Here, we aim to provide a general conceptualization of leishmaniasis by summarizing the historical development of the disease to provide a better understanding for possible future approaches.

2. History of the disease

In 1885, after observing *Leishmania* organism for the first time, Cunningham stated that the organism was not a bacteria. Thirteen years later, a Russian military surgeon Peter Borovsky further found out that the organism was a protozoan which was also confirmed by Wright in 1903. During that time, William Leishman and Charles Donovan described the agent responsible from VL. Leishman conducting his study in India observed enlargement of the spleen and fever in patients which he further observed the samples he took from the patients under the microscope using Romanowsky method for staining and stated that it was not like anything he had seen before [13]. Finally, in 1942, female phlebotomine sandflies had enough evidence to be accepted as the main vector for CL and VL due to the fact that clinical conditions observed following a sandfly bite described as histiocytoses [14]. In terms of changing face of diagnosis of leishmaniasis, starting from the microscopical identification of the agents, medical technologies have progressed in time further into PCR-based DNA sequencing methods for determination of specific species.

L. donovani was the first identified *Leishmania* species taking its name from William Leishman and Charles Donovan which was given by Ross in order to give credit to their studies [15].

Despite being a neglected tropical disease, our knowledge about the disease has been increasing continuously. Case reports involving uncommon laryngeal leishmaniasis- and HIV-infected individuals showing leishmaniasis effects such as skin lesions and nodules have shown that leishmaniasis can occur again even after treatment hinting to the incubation period of parasite (**Figure 1**) [16, 17].

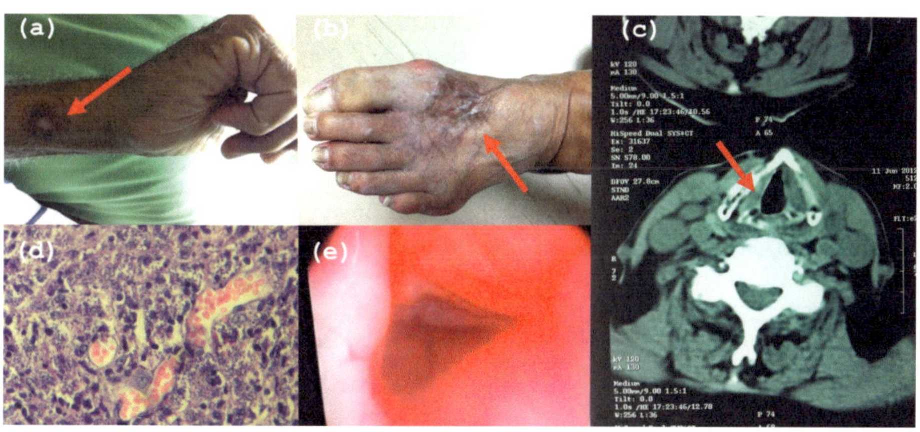

Figure 1.
A rare case of treated laryngeal ML which originated from a previous CL of hands and feet. Isolated agent is L. infantum in this 81-year-old male patient resident in Adana, Turkey, a subtropical area. (a) CL lesions on a patients hand on his first application to clinic. (b) CL lesions on patients foot on his first application to clinic. (c) BT of neck showing papillomatous push elongating into ventricles. (d) Histological examination of laryngeal biopsy specimen (May-Grunwald-Giemsa staining; original magnification, ×1000) showing intracellular amastigotes of Leishmania species and histiocytes with vacuolated cytoplasm and corpuscles inside. (e) Laryngoscopic examination showing lesions with edema and erythema due to ML. Reprinted from [16].

Treatment of leishmaniasis started with the use of pentavalent antimonials in the 1940s. Parasite gaining resistance and high level of toxicity for these drugs made it necessary to find an alternative. Amphotericin B is an alternative drug that has been in use since 1980. The main action mechanism of amphotericin B is to interfere with the membrane lipids and cause disruption. The length of the therapy changes between 15 and 45 days for different cases, whereas dosage can vary. Combinatorial use of this drug with some other drugs has shown great increase in the effectiveness of treatment.

3. Epidemiology

Leishmaniasis is a globally common disease that affects more than 98 countries and territories. Even though its effects are mainly observed in underdeveloped or developing countries, this parasite has spread to Europe and the United States due to the traveling to these areas and immigration from these areas. Old World leishmaniasis is endemic in Asia, Africa, the Mediterranean, and the Middle East. *L. tropica*, *L. major*, *Leishmania aethiopica*, and *L. donovani* are the four common species causing Old World leishmaniasis. New World leishmaniasis is caused by the *Leishmania mexicana*, *Leishmania braziliensis*, and *Leishmania guyanensis*. In total, six Old World countries (Afghanistan, Algeria, Arabian Peninsula, Syria, Sudan, and Iran) and two New World countries (Brazil and Peru) make up 90% of all leishmaniasis reports [18].

Poor process of record taking in underdeveloped and developing countries makes it difficult to determine its incidence and prevalence in certain areas. Syria is reported to have highest amount of incidence in the Middle East with 52,983 cases being reported in 2012 [19]. In Iraq, leishmaniasis had a prevalence of 45.5 cases per 100,000 of population in 1992 due to the war and population migration which can give an estimate of current situation [19].

In Asia, Afghanistan, Iran, and Syria are the three Middle Eastern countries where CL is endemic and reported most. Syria having the most amount of CL cases also named the disease as Aleppo boil [20]. Moving toward Eastern Asia, Pakistan holds great number of CL cases, whereas India and Bangladesh can be considered as the sole reservoir for VL [7]. In China, there are three defined VL types: anthroponotic VL, which is caused by *L. donovani*; zoonotic mountain-type zoonotic VL; and zoonotic desert-type VL in which both are caused by *L. Infantum* [21]. Depending on the habitat, there are four vectors when it comes to VL transmission in China [21]: *Phlebotomus chinensis* and *Phlebotomus longiductus* for anthroponotic VL in domiciliary habitats, *P. chinensis* for mountain-type zoonotic VL in wild and peridomestic habitats, and *Phlebotomus wui* and *Phlebotomus alexandri* for zoonotic desert-type VL in wild habitats [21].

In Africa, three *Leishmania* species, *L. infantum*, *L. major*, and *L. tropica*, are responsible from the CL cases [8]. Egypt, Algeria, Morocco, Tunisia, and Libya are the Northern African countries with the highest amount of reported CL cases between 2003 and 2009 [7]. Among East Africa, countries such as Ethiopia, Sudan, and Somalia have highest number of reported VL cases between years 2004 and 2009, which contribute to a large portion of total amount of 8569 cases in the region [7]. In Cameroon, survey done in Mokolo region consisting of 32,466 people showed 146 active CL lesions and 261 people having scars probably as a result of prior CL infection [22]. Interestingly, it was also noted that 4.8% of the patients with CL observed to be positive for HIV infection [22].

Realizing the importance of leishmaniasis in most of the African countries is a challenge compared to other countries because of the low quality healthcare services, poor data management, and absent reports. East Africa and sub-Saharan Africa are the geographical regions where leishmaniasis was the least common until 2012 [7]. Considering leishmaniasis is endemic in these regions, it is safe to say that observed value will be much different than the real outcome once enough data are gathered.

When it comes to Europe, countries in the Mediterranean region such as Italy, Greece, Turkey, and Albania have highest prevalence of VL cases [7]. In addition, few number of VL cases were observed in France, Spain, Portugal, and Croatia [7]. In terms of CL cases, Turkey holds great percentage of reports compared to others. In the Netherlands, 185 CL, 8 VL, and 2 MCL cases were observed between 2005 and 2012 [23]. In general, traveling to endemic regions such as Afghanistan or Morocco is shown as a significant risk factor of *Leishmania* cases in developed countries. Due to the nature of leishmaniasis infection, developed European countries have low amount of reported cases, and in most of the cases, insufficient immune system is the other most important risk factor in addition to trips to endemic regions [24].

American region has low VL and high amount of CL cases reported in general with a 1–20 difference. Brazil has the highest amount of reported cases both in VL and CL. Colombia, Peru, Nicaragua, and Venezuela are other areas where CL cases happen frequently [7].

Mexico, the United States, and Canada have relatively low amount of reported cases in terms of global occurrence. A total of 811 CL and 7 VL cases were reported in Mexico between 2004 and 2008. The US Army Forces going to endemic regions such as Afghanistan for military duty resulted in few reported *Leishmania* cases in the United States.

Australia and Antarctica are the two continents where leishmaniasis is not considered to be endemic [2]. Between the years 2008 and 2014, 52 CL and 3 VL cases were reported in Australia [25]. Traveling to *Leishmania* parasite endemic regions is thought to be the reason for most of these cases as similar with the cases seen in Europe [25]. *L. tropica* was identified in 30 patients and was the highest compared to 4 other identified species [25].

4. Transmission and prevention

Only vector responsible for transmitting leishmaniasis is the female sandfly, belonging to the genera *Phlebotomus* spp. in the Old World and *Lutzomyia* spp. in the New World [3]. Out of the many known sandfly species, 93 of them are known to spread leishmaniasis. Sandflies are usually active during night time, and they have limited ability to move. They are usually 2 mm large and are capable of tearing the skin in order to feed on blood. Mainly observed in the tropical regions, they have spread to the Northern European regions due to the increasing temperatures and climate changes.

Transmission can be zoonotic or anthroponotic depending on the reservoir. Domestic dogs are considered to be the major reservoir for zoonotic transmission. In the Americas and Central Asia, interaction between wild animals and humans also causes zoonotic transmission. Humans with VL or post kala-azar dermal leishmaniasis serve as the only reservoir in anthroponotic transmission.

Attenuated parasite vaccines that will provide long-term immunity and prevent transmission are in development. Zoonotic transmission occurs with dogs, and treatment methods targeting infected dogs are not preferred due to the fact that it may result with increased resistance for parasite or there is a high chance of infection in the nature even after the treatment [6]. Deltamethrin-treated collars were tested for the control of the disease and a significant reduction in infection levels in dogs was observed [6]. Avoiding outdoor areas in endemic areas, using protective clothing, using insect repellents, covering around the bed with a net, sleeping above the ground level, and avoiding night time activities are some of the useful methods in order to prevent transmission in humans.

5. Host-parasite interactions

Once *Leishmania* enters the human host, macrophages try to attack *Leishmania* with reactive oxygen and nitrogen molecules. *Leishmania* parasite produces protease with increased activity which considerably lowers macrophage activity. Inside the cell, phagosomes consume the parasite, but they are ineffective against the parasite as a result of parasite changing the destructive properties of phagosome.

Protective immune response to leishmaniasis mainly depends on the T-cell subset response accompanied with the specific cytokines, transcription factors, presenting of antigen, and production of various interleukins having direct or indirect effect on the main immune system. However, it is important to note that susceptibility or resistance to leishmaniasis is possible in individuals with altered genetics or depending on the environmental conditions as well as parasite strain starting the infection [26].

Immune response starts with the cells of innate immune system. Neutrophils are the first immune system cells responding to the sandfly bite starting the leishmaniasis infection [27]. Neutrophils are capable of producing microbicidal factors effective against *Leishmania* such as nitric oxide (NO) and neutrophil extracellular traps [27, 28]. Neutrophils are effective protective agent in most forms of the leishmaniasis, but this is usually affected by the host genetics and *Leishmania* strain effecting the host [27]. Neutral killers are also recruited to the site of infection after neutrophils, and their cytotoxic activity is effective against parasite by mediating lysis [29, 30]. Organ-specific protection during the early stages of infection is the case for natural killer T cells [31]. Increased natural killer T-cell concentration during the disease progress and decreased concentration following treatment indicates importance in early response [32]. T cells also play an important role in immune response. Nitric oxide production in order to fight with the parasite is induced by IFN-γ-producing Th1 cells [27]. However, Th2 is responsible from the susceptibility because of its ability to produce cytokines such as IL-4 and IL-13 [27]. The regulatory T cells maintain a critical role in IL-10 expression and continuity of parasite immunity [27, 33].

Leishmania parasites have developed their own way in order to reduce the effectiveness of immune system. Modifying toll-like receptors' pathogen recognition ability, delaying phagosomes ability to terminate parasite once consumed, altering macrophage antigen presentation, and modifying host signaling in order to effect production or inhibition of certain cytokines or chemokines such as IL-10 and IL-12 are some of the examples of immune evasion mechanisms used by parasites [27]. Being a progressive disease, increased concentrations of IFN-γ and TNF-α cytokines indicate immunosuppressive mechanism for leishmaniasis especially in VL [34–37]. IL-10, which is produced by many immune system cells such as B cells, T-cell subsets, and innate cells, is a regulatory cytokine responsible from immune suppression and reducing the effectiveness of antigen-presenting cells like macrophages and dendritic cells where initial response mainly depends on this process [34]. For VL, IL-10 was found to be majorly produced by CD4 + CD25-Foxp3- cells in the spleen suggesting that suppression of antileishmanial immunity in effected individuals depends on the expression of IL-10 by T cells. In addition, experiments done with mouse models have shown that IL-12 signaling and presence of high antigen dose can lead to the activation of Th1 cells which coexpresses IL-10 [38]. IL-27 is another immune system regulator which promotes T cells to produce IL-10 following an infection [39]. Furthermore, upregulation of IL-21 by T cells in order to reach elevated levels of IL-10 is thought to be the role of IL-27 [40]. In order to determine immune system cells responsible from the production of IL-10 and IL-27, splenic aspirate cells obtained from the VL spleen was tested for expression levels of mRNA for various cells. CD14+ cells were found to be main source of IL-27-related mRNA expression, whereas CD3+ T cells were the main source of both IL-10 and IL-21 [40]. For CL, mouse models showed that IL-22 plays a critical role in the progression of pathology such that increased levels of IL-22 help maintain skin integrity and prevent further inflammation [41].

IFN-γ is another important immune system molecule produced by parasite-dependent Th1 CD4+ lymphocytes and is related to intracellular control of parasites upon infection. On the other hand, Th2 CD4+ cells are responsible from the progression of the disease. This difference in Th1 and Th2 cell line responses was further confirmed by Holaday et al.'s study done on mouse models carrying specific mutations. The study showed that in the presence of antigen, Th1-like cell line response was to produce IL-2 and IFN-γ, whereas Th2-like cell line response was to produce IL-4 and IL-5 upon stimulation [42].

In another study, Th1, Th2, and Th17 CD4+ T-cell subsets were found to induce production of IL-10 despite having different signaling pathways and transcription route. ERK1 and ERK2 transcriptional activation was common in all these Th cell subsets. c-Maf is an important transcription factor in macrophages for the process of IL-10 expression and was also found to be common for the previously mentioned three different T-cell subsets. c-Maf expression was also found to be dependent on ERK activation in Th1 and Th17 cells [38].

6. Clinical characteristics of the disease in humans

Cutaneous leishmaniasis is the milder form of leishmaniasis and usually leads to formation of skin lesions or nodules around the exposed bite sites such as face, neck, or limbs [8, 24]. Lesions can heal spontaneously in few months, or in some extreme cases, it can take few years to resolve [8]. Although CL is self-curing and nonlife-threatening, accumulation of CL often leads to disfigured formations on skin. Lesion number can vary between 1 and 20, and upon healing, distinct scars are left on the skin. Various treatment methods are used in order to speed up the healing process for CL.

Depending on the disease forms observed clinically such as uncomplicated form, chronic recurrent form, and diffuse form, there are four causative pathogens in the Old World and five causative pathogens in the New World [18]. *L. major*, *L. tropica*, *L. infantum*, and *L. aethiopica* are the pathogens of Old World, whereas *L. L. mexicana*, *L. L. amazonensis*, *L. V. braziliensis*, *L. V. guyanensis*, and *L. V. panamensis* are the pathogens of New World in the case of CL [18].

VL also known as kala-azar is the fatal form of leishmaniasis with a mortality rate of 75–95%. Macrophages affected by the parasite spread the infection throughout the body, and patients develop pancytopenia and immunosuppression [6, 43, 44]. VL is often discussed together with HIV as they both affect immune system heavily making patients susceptible to other infections. Incubation period is between 2 weeks and 2 years. Liver- and spleen-related problems are common in patients with VL.

Parasite spreading around the initial bite site using the lymphatic way and infecting the nose or mouth mucosa leads to ML (**Figure 1**) [45]. Immune system reacting to parasite at the tip of the nose effects airway walls causing lumen obstruction which is related to necrosis of the cartilage in the nose. Unlike CL, ML is not a self-healing disease and can cause permanent skin problems. Destruction of the tip of the nose is a severe condition that may affect patients in their social life. Breathing problems are common result of ML in patients due to the blocked airways [46].

Another form of the disease, post kala-azar dermal leishmaniasis is a complication of VL in which patients cured of VL develops nodular, macular, or maculopapular rash on skin as a result of immune suppression following VL. It is mainly observed in Sudan and India where majority of the VL cases progress into post kala-azar dermal leishmaniasis [47].

7. Treatment and resistance in humans

There are various treatment methods depending on the host immune system effectiveness and the type of *Leishmania* effecting the host as well as the way parasite is transmitted. Host factors such as genetics or immune response or factors related to treatment such as dosage, duration, and completion of the therapy and finally factors related to the parasite, such as intrinsic sensitivity of the species and lack of resistance to the medication are important determinants regarding to treatment of the disease. Long incubation period of *Leishmania* parasite makes it a challenge in detection and early treatment methods. If applicable early treatment should be applied in order to further prevent the spreading of the parasite. Having no effective human vaccines puts the disease at a critical point.

Pentavalent antimonials, sodium stibogluconate and N-methylglucamine, liposomal amphotericin B, miltefosine, and paramycin are some of the widely used drugs in routine treatment [6, 48]. Compared to liposomal amphotericin B which is a less toxic form, conventional amphotericin B has complicated application procedure and harmful side effects making liposomal amphotericin B a better choice in treatment of both CL and VL which is also an antifungal agent. Still in some underdeveloped or developing countries that cannot afford liposomal amphotericin B treatment, pentavalent antimonials are used. Despite their toxic effects on the liver and kidneys, pentavalent antimonials are still highly effective [49]. On the other hand, emerging resistance limits the therapy frequently. Miltefosine is another drug with known effect of inducing parasite resistance if not used properly.

Global antibiotic resistance problem has emerged in the treatment of leishmaniasis too, and a number of papers reporting treatment failures are increasing [50]. Anthroponotic transmission is the main cause of drug resistance in *Leishmania* species. Humans being the anthroponotic host, various effects can lead to drug resistance for parasite once treatment starts. Ignoring the recommended consuming amount and frequency of the drug, reduced concentration of the drug effecting the parasite, inhibition of drug activation, inactivation of active drug, and alterations in host gene amplifications are some important example mechanisms for parasites gaining drug resistance. Although, the mechanisms of drug resistance in *Leishmania* species are not well elucidated in detail, but the involvement of P-glycoprotein (Pgp)-like ABC transporters and ldmdr1 gene has been detected in hard-to-treat parasites [51–54]. In addition, high amount of thiol levels was found to play a role in developing resistance as they prevent reduction of pentavalent antimonials to trivalent antimonials [55].

8. Latest developments in the diagnosis, prevention, and treatment

Permanent solution for the leishmaniasis in terms of successful human vaccination is still a major challenge. However, there are different vaccinations currently being tested in mouse model. One of them uses "killed but metabolically active" parasites to induce host immune system reaction. Mice infected by "killed but metabolically active" *L. infantum chagasi* showed no signs of organomegaly or parasite presence 6 months after infection compared to mice infected with live parasite. Finally "killed but metabolically active" *L. infantum chagasi* has also shown to induce parasite-specific protective host immune response that is similar to response induced by live *Leishmania* [56].

Using salivary peptides of the sandfly holds potential to be used as a vaccine component; however, complex immune response makes it a challenge. Novel drug combinations have been tested in some endemic regions in order to lower the treatment cost and toxicity and preventing resistance gain by the parasite. Nitroquinolines were found to show leishmanicidal activity. Antimicrobial peptides including dermaseptin, andropin, and cecropin have been found effective against CL. Edelfosine is an oral drug with greatly increased activity compared to miltefosine. There are also compounds isolated from plants which are tested and observed to have antileishmanial activity. For example, a polyphenolic flavanoid, quercetin, has shown antileishmanial activity in treatment of VL [57]. Four plant species named *Agave americana*, *Azadirachta indica*, *Eclipta alba*, and *Piper longum* showed important antileishmanial activity too [58–61].

Macrophage targeted drug delivery system is another novel approach to directly effect *Leishmania* parasites that live in the macrophages as their infection mechanism. As getting into macrophages is a challenge, liposomes, microspheres, nanoparticles, and carbon nanotubes are some of the various drug carriers that are studied to target macrophages [62]. In addition, use of specific receptors expressed by macrophages to actively deliver a drug is also used [63].

9. Conclusion and future perspectives

Leishmaniasis still remains as a big public health challenge in some parts of the world. Despite developments in scientific knowledge and medical technology, there is still a need for quick and cheap detection of *Leishmania* infections especially in endemic areas. Studies focusing on molecular microbiological methods can help to develop new diagnostic methods.

In terms of treatment of leishmaniasis, emerging resistance is a big threat for infectious disease specialists like in other microbial diseases. There are two arms of fight. One is the development of a successful vaccine, and the other is the progress of finding new compounds to cure the infection. If applicable early treatment should be applied in order to further prevent the spreading of the parasite. Having no effective human vaccines puts the disease at this critical point. That is why studies focusing on the development of vaccine will be pathfinder in the future decade. On the other hand, studies evaluating the antileishmanial activity of various natural products or chemically modified compounds are needed to find new opportunities in successful treatment of *Leishmania* infections for the future.

Acknowledgements

The author wants to express his special thanks to Namık Refik Kerküklü for his kind help during the preperation of this chapter.

Author details

Mümtaz Güran
Faculty of Medicine, Eastern Mediterranean University, Famagusta, Turkey

*Address all correspondence to: mumtaz.guran@emu.edu.tr

IntechOpen

References

[1] Akbari M, Oryan A, Hatam G. Application of nanotechnology in treatment of leishmaniasis: A review. Acta Tropica. 2017;**172**:86-90

[2] Handler MZ, Patel PA, Kapila R, Al-Qubati Y, Schwartz RA. Cutaneous and mucocutaneous leishmaniasis: Clinical perspectives. Journal of the American Academy of Dermatology. 2015;**73**(6):897-908

[3] Pace D. Leishmaniasis. The Journal of Infection. 2014;**69**(S1):S10-S18

[4] Di Muccio T et al. Epidemiology of imported leishmaniasis in Italy: Implications for a European endemic country. PLoS ONE. 2015;**10**(6):1-16

[5] Antinori S, Gianelli E, Calattini S, Longhi E, Gramiccia M, Corbellino M. Cutaneous leishmaniasis: An increasing threat for travellers. Clinical Microbiology and Infection. 2005;**11**(5):343-346

[6] Oryan A, Akbari M. Worldwide risk factors in leishmaniasis. Asian Pacific Journal of Tropical Medicine. 2016;**9**(10):925-932

[7] Alvar J et al. Leishmaniasis worldwide and global estimates of its incidence. PLoS ONE. 2012;**7**(5):e35671

[8] Mohammadi MA, Bamorovat M, FasihiHarandi M, Karimi T, Sharifi I, Aflatoonian MR. Comparison of three PCR-based methods for simplicity and cost effectiveness identification of cutaneous leishmaniasis due to Leishmaniatropica. Iranian Journal of Parasitology. 2017;**12**(2):215-223

[9] Bates PA. Transmission of Leishmaniametacyclicpromastigotes by phlebotomine sand flies. International Journal for Parasitology. 2007;**37**(10):1097-1106

[10] Ready PD. Sand fly evolution and its relationship to Leishmania transmission. Memórias do Instituto Oswaldo Cruz. 2000;**95**(4):589-590

[11] Ready PD. Leishmaniasis emergence in Europe. Eurosurveillance. 2010;**15**(10):29-39

[12] Ribeiro PAF et al. Evaluation of a Leishmania hypothetical protein administered as DNA vaccine or recombinant protein against Leishmaniainfantum infection and its immunogenicity in humans. Cellular Immunology. 2018;**331**:67-77

[13] Leishman WB. On the possibility of the occurrence of trypanosomiasis in India. British Medical Journal. 1903;**2**(2238):1376-1377

[14] Gotoff SP, Esterly NB. Histiocytosis. The Journal of Pediatrics. 1 Oct 1974; **85**(4):592-594

[15] Ross MR. Further notes on leishman's bodies. British Medical Journal. 1903;**2**(2239):1401

[16] Gökmen TG, Haytoglu S, Güran M, Kusçu F, Köksal F. A multidisciplinary approach to an uncommon case of laryngeal leishmaniasis in Turkey. Journal of Vector Borne Diseases. 2014;**51**(2):140-143

[17] Barroso DH, Silva CEF, e Vasconcelos ACDP, Cavalcanti SM d M, de Brito MEF, Medeiros ACR. Post-kala-azar dermal leishmaniasis in two different clinical contexts. Anais Brasileiros de Dermatologia. 2015;**90**(3):108-110

[18] Von Stebut E. Leishmaniasis. Journal der Deutschen Dermatologischen Gesellschaft. 2015;**13**(3):191-201

[19] Salam N, Al-Shaqha WM, Azzi A. Leishmaniasis in the middle East: Incidence and epidemiology. *PLoS Neglected Tropical Diseases*. 2014;**8**(10):1-8

[20] Rioux J, Jalouk L, Khiami A, Ilaboratoire CD. Evidence for a

long-term Aleppo, Syria increase in the incidence of Leishmania Tropica in Aleppo, Syria. Transactions of the Royal Society of Tropical Medicine and Hygiene. 1993;**87**(3):247-249

[21] Lun ZR et al. Visceral leishmaniasis in China: An endemic disease under control. Clinical Microbiology Reviews. 2015;**28**(4):987-1004

[22] Ngouateu OB et al. Clinical features and epidemiology of cutaneous leishmaniasis and Leishmania major/ HIV co-infection in Cameroon: Results of a large cross-sectional study. Transactions of the Royal Society of Tropical Medicine and Hygiene. 2012;**106**(3):137-142

[23] Bart A, van Thiel PP, de Vries HJ, Hodiamont CJ, Van Gool T. Imported leishmaniasisin the Netherlands from 2005 to 2012: Epidemiology, diagnostic techniques and sequence-based species typing from 195 patients. Eurosurveillance. 2013;**18**(30)

[24] Pigott DM, Bhatt S, Golding N, et al. Global distribution maps of the leishmaniases. Elife. 27 Jun 2014;**3**:e02851

[25] Roberts T et al. Molecular epidemiology of imported cases of leishmaniasis in Australia from 2008 to 2014. PLoS ONE. 2015;**10**(3):1-11

[26] Kumar R, Nylén S. Immunobiology of visceral leishmaniasis. Frontiers in Immunology. 2012;**3**:1-10

[27] Gupta G, Oghumu S, Satoskar AR. Mechanisms of immune evasion inLeishmaniasis. Advances in Applied Microbiology. 2014;**82**:1-23

[28] Guimaraes-Costa AB et al. Leishmaniaamazonensispromastigotes induce and are killed by neutrophil extracellular traps. Proceedings of the National Academy of Sciences. 2009;**106**(16):6748-6753

[29] Lieke T, Nyln S, Eidsmo L, Schmetz C, Berg L, Akuffo H. The interplay between Leishmaniapromastigotes and human natural killer cells in vitro leads to direct lysis of Leishmania by NK cells and modulation of NK cell activity by Leishmaniapromastigotes. Parasitology. 2011;**138**(14):1898-1909

[30] Thalhofer CJ, Chen Y, Sudan B, Love-Homan L, Wilson ME. Leukocytes infiltrate the skin and draining lymph nodes in response to the protozoan leishmaniainfantumchagasi. Infection and Immunity. 2011;**79**(1):108-117

[31] Mattner J, Donhauser N, Werner-Felmayer G, Bogdan C. NKT cells mediate organ-specific resistance against Leishmania major infection. Microbes and Infection. 2006;**8**(2):354-362

[32] Rai AK, Thakur CP, Seth T, Mitra DK. Enrichment of invariant natural killer T cells in the bone marrow of visceral leishmaniasis patients. Parasite Immunology. 2011;**33**(12):688-691

[33] Belkaid Y, Piccirillo CA, Mendez S. CD4+ CD25+ regulatory T cells control Leishmania major persistence and immunity, Nature, vol. 420, no.September, 2002. pp. 633-637

[34] Ansari NA, Saluja S, Salotra P. Elevated levels of interferon-γ, interleukin-10, and interleukin-6 during active disease in Indian kalaazar. Clinical Immunology. 2006;**119**(3):339-345

[35] Caldas A et al. Balance of IL-10 and interferon-γ plasma levels in human visceral leishmaniasis: Implications in the pathogenesis. BMC Infectious Diseases. 2005;**5**:1-9

[36] Ghalib HW, Ahmed M, Steven G. Interleukin 10 production correlates with pathology in human Leishmania

donovani infections. Journal of Clinical Investigation. 1993;**92**:324-329

[37] Karp CL et al. In vivo cytokine profiles in patients with kala-azar. The Journal of Clinical Investigation. 1993;**91**:1644-1648

[38] Saraiva M, Christensen JR, Veldhoen M, Murphy TL, Murphy KM, O'Garra A. Interleukin-10 production by Th1 cells requires interleukin-12-induced STAT4 transcription factor and ERK MAP kinase activation by high antigen dose. Immunity. 2009;**31**(2):209-219

[39] Stumhofer JS et al. Interleukins 27 and 6 induce STAT3-mediated T cell production of interleukin 10. Nature Immunology. 2007;**8**(12):1363-1371

[40] Prajapati VK et al. Targeted killing of leishmaniadonovani in vivo and in vitro with amphotericin β attached to functionalized carbon nanotubes. The Journal of Antimicrobial Chemotherapy. 2011;**66**(4):874-879

[41] Gimblet C et al. IL-22 protects against tissue damage during cutaneous leishmaniasis. PLoS ONE. 2015;**10**(8):1-18

[42] Holaday BJ, Sadick MD, Wang ZE, et al. Reconstitution of Leishmania immunity in severe combined immunodeficient mice using Th1-and Th2-like cell lines. The Journal of Immunology. 1 Sep 1991;**147**(5):1653-1658

[43] Nozzi M, Del Torto M, Chiarelli F, Breda L. Leishmaniasis and autoimmune diseases in pediatric age. Cellular Immunology. 2014;**292**(1):9-13

[44] Mcgwire BS, Satoskar AR. Leishmaniasis: Clinical syndromes and treatment. QJM. 2014;**107**(1):7-14

[45] Mansueto P, Seidita A, Vitale G, Cascio A. Leishmaniasis in travelers: A literature review. Travel Medicine and Infectious Disease. 2014;**12**(6):563-581

[46] Mans DR, Kent AD, Hu RVPF, Schallig HD. Epidemiological, biological and clinical aspects of Leishmaniasis with special emphasis on BusiYasi in Suriname. Journal of Clinical and Experimental Dermatology Research. 2017;**08**(02):388

[47] Faleiro RJ, Kumar R, Hafner LM, Engwerda CR. Immune regulation during chronic visceral Leishmaniasis. PLoS Neglected Tropical Diseases. 2014;**8**(7):e2914

[48] Anversa L et al. Human leishmaniasis in Brazil: A general review. Revista da Associação Médica Brasileira. 2018;**64**(3):281-289

[49] Croft S, Yardley V. Chemotherapy of leishmaniasis. Current Pharmaceutical Design. 2002;**8**(4):319-342

[50] Mondelaers A, Hendrickx S, Van Bockstal L, Maes L, Caljon G. Miltefosine-resistant Leishmaniainfantum strains with an impaired MT/ROS3 transporter complex retain amphotericin B susceptibility. The Journal of Antimicrobial Chemotherapy. 2017;**73**(2):392-394

[51] Socolsky C, Salamanca E, Gimenez A, Borkosky SA, Bardon A. Prenylatedacylphloroglucinolswith Leishmanicidalactivity from the fern elaphoglossumlindbergii. Journal of Natural Products. Jan. 2016;**79**(1):98-105

[52] Manzano JI, García-Hernández R, Castanys S, Gamarro F. A new ABC half-transporter in Leishmania major is involved in resistance to antimony. Antimicrobial Agents and Chemotherapy. 2013;**57**(8):3719-3730

[53] Henderson DM, Sifri CD, Rodgers M, Wirth DF, Hendrickson N, Ullman B. Multidrug resistance in Leishmaniadonovani is conferred by amplification of a gene homologous to the mammalian mdr1 gene.

Molecular and Cellular Biology. Jun. 1992;**12**(6):2855-2865

[54] Tanwar J, Das S, Fatima Z, Hameed S. Multidrug resistance: An emerging crisis. Interdisciplinary Perspectives on Infectious Diseases. 2014;**2014**:541340

[55] Mohapatra S. Drug resistance in leishmaniasis: Newer developments. Tropical Parasitology. 2014;**4**(1):4

[56] Bruhn KW et al. Killed but metabolically active Leishmaniainfantum as a novel whole-cell vaccine for visceral leishmaniasis. Clinical and Vaccine Immunology. 2012;**19**(4):490-498

[57] Da Silva ER, Maquiaveli C d C, Magalhães PP. The leishmanicidalflavonolsquercetin and quercitrin target Leishmania (Leishmania) amazonensisarginase. Experimental Parasitology. 2012;**130**(3):183-188

[58] Thakur CP et al. Anti-leishmanial activity of Agave Americana L.–A traditional Indian medicinal plant. Indian Journal of Traditional Knowledge. 2015;**14**(4):658-663

[59] Carneiro SMP, Carvalho FAA, Santana LCLR, Sousa APL, Neto JMM, Chaves MH. The cytotoxic and antileishmanial activity of extracts and fractions of leaves and fruits of Azadirachtaindica (aJuss.). Biological Research. 2012;**45**(2):111-116

[60] Khanna VG, Kannabiran K, Getti G. Leishmanicidal activity of saponins isolated from the leaves of Ecliptaprostrata and Gymnemasylvestre. Indian Journal of Pharmacology. 2009;**41**(1):32-35

[61] Chouhan G et al. Leishmanicidal activity of Piper nigrum bioactive fractions is interceded via apoptosis in vitro and substantiated by Th1 immunostimulatory potential in vivo. Frontiers in Microbiology. 2015;**6**:1-19

[62] de Souza A et al. Promising nanotherapy in treating leishmaniasis. International Journal of Pharmaceutics. 2018;**547**(1-2):421-431

[63] Jain K, Jain NK. Novel therapeutic strategies for treatment of visceral leishmaniasis. Drug Discovery Today. 2013;**18**(23-24):1272-1281

Chapter 6

Vector-Borne Infections in Bulgaria

Iva Christova

Abstract

Bulgaria is an endemic country for Lyme borreliosis and Crimean-Congo hemorrhagic fever (CCHF). Sporadic cases of tick-borne encephalitis (TBE) and West Nile virus (WNV) encephalitis have been also reported. The reported incidence of Lyme borreliosis in Bulgaria is about 6/100,000 population. Two peaks in the seasonal distribution of cases and more frequent presentation of neuroborreliosis than of Lyme arthritis appear to be characteristics of Lyme borreliosis in Bulgaria. *Borrelia afzelii* is highly prevalent in Bulgarian *Ixodes ricinus* ticks. With sporadic cases or small outbreaks, CCHF appeared every year since the 1950s. For the last 10 years, a total of 60 CCHF cases were officially recorded. There is a tendency for CCHF to spread in previously non-endemic areas. The strains causing CCHF in the country belong to lineage Europe 1. A mean of 3.7% CCHF seroprevalence among the Bulgarian population is established. Both Europe 1 and Europe 2 CCHF virus lineages are present in ticks in Bulgaria. Tick-borne encephalitis (TBE) is very unusual. Only a few cases of TBE have been detected. Overall seroprevalence of 0.6% for TBE virus was found in humans. In 2015, a few WNV human cases were detected caused by lineage 2. Overall WNV seroprevalence in human population in the country is 1.5%.

Keywords: TBE, CCHF, WNV, Lyme borreliosis

1. Lyme borreliosis

1.1 Introduction

Lyme borreliosis is the most prevalent tick-borne infection in the North hemisphere. It is a chronic and multisystem infectious disease caused by several species of *Borrelia burgdorferi* sensu lato complex. Three main species are known to cause the disease in Europe, namely *Borrelia afzelii*, *Borrelia garinii*, and *Borrelia burgdorferi* sensu stricto. The ability to cause persistent infection in humans and a wide variety of mammalian hosts is a common property of Lyme disease.

Early manifestations of Lyme disease include typical skin lesion erythema migrans as a sign of early localized infection and/or unspecific flu-like symptoms, acute meningitis or meningopolyneuritis, and acute arthritis, which are signs of early disseminated infection. Late manifestations may appear as chronic neurological abnormalities, chronic arthritis, or acrodermatitis chronica atrophicans, marking late disseminated infection.

Bulgaria is endemic for Lyme borreliosis and a country with mandatory notification of the disease. The reported incidence of Lyme borreliosis in Bulgaria is about 6/100,000 of the population, but the true incidence is most probably much higher, because the disease often is self-limited and mild cases go unrecognized.

IntechOpen

1.2 Clinical features of Lyme borreliosis in humans in Bulgaria

Bulgarian study on clinical manifestations of 1257 patients with Lyme borreliosis, diagnosed by physicians and confirmed in laboratory (except for erythema migrans), showed that the most common clinical presentation is erythema migrans (EM), diagnosed in 868 (69.1%) of the patients, almost uniformly as a sole presentation and rarely as a part of multisystem involvement. Rashes had a median diameter of 11 cm (5–35 cm). The erythema rash was homogenous in 44% and with central clearing and peripheral border in 56%. In 14.7% of the patients, atypical rashes with a vesicular or ulcerated center were found. Flu-like symptoms, such as fever, headache, myalgia, arthralgia, fatigue, neck stiffness, were the most common signs associated with EM. Fever was found on physical examination in 133 (15.3%) of the EM patients. In parallel with EM, lymphadenopathy was detected in 284 (32.7%) of the EM cases. In addition, multiple EM was detected in 59 (6.8%) of the patients.

After EM, the second most frequent presentation of Lyme disease in Bulgaria is neuroborreliosis. It is usually presented as radiculoneuritis as a sole presentation (found in 72% of the patients with neuroborreliosis in Bulgaria) and much rarely manifested as cranial neuritis (mainly in children), myelitis, meningoradiculoneuritis, or encephalopathy.

The third most common presentation of Lyme disease in Bulgaria is Lyme arthritis. In the same study, it was diagnosed in 101 (8%) of the patients with Lyme borreliosis. Lyme arthritis was mainly presented by brief attacks of arthritis and rarely as chronic arthritis.

Rare manifestations of Lyme borreliosis in Bulgaria are those affecting heart and eyes (found in 1.1 and 0.9%, respectively). Very rare syndromes are borrelial lymphocytoma and acrodermatitis chronica atrophicans (0.3%).

Multiple organ involvement was found in 2.1% of the patients. Most commonly it was presented as neurological disorders and skin lesions or arthritis.

In addition, the highest proportion of the patients with Lyme borreliosis is in children aged 5–9. The disease shows two peaks in the seasonal distribution of the cases. Neuroborreliosis is a more frequent presentation than Lyme arthritis in Bulgaria.

1.3 Borrelial C6 peptides as antigens for serological diagnosis of Lyme borreliosis

Diagnosis of Lyme borreliosis depends on clinical signs supported by serological findings—enzyme-linked immunosorbent assay (ELISA) and immunoblotting. Various *B. burgdorferi* sensu lato protein antigens are used for ELISA tests (OspA, OspC, FlaB, VlsE). VlsE is the most promising diagnostic antigen among them due to the conserved immunogenic epitopes.

VlsE gene consists of expression site and 15 silent cassettes with a high degree of homology and high rate of reassortments. Each cassette consists of six variable and six invariable regions. The 26-amino-acid-long sixth invariable region (IR6) is immunodominant and much conserved among *B. burgdorferi* sensu lato species. It was shown that IgG antibodies to IR6 (C6) are often detected in early and late Lyme borreliosis [1, 2]. These two statements, i.e. that C6: (1) possess high immunogenicity and (2) is highly conserved among species of the complex B. burgdorferi sensu lato, we decided to test in practice with serum samples from Bulgarian patients with Lyme disease.

Four 26-amino-acid-long peptides were synthesized (ProteoGenix SAS, France), which corresponded to IR6 regions of VlsE proteins from *B. burgdorferi* sensu stricto, *B. garinii*, and *B. afzelii*. Because of the previously described difference in reactivity [1], two peptides were synthesized from two strains of *B. burgdorferi* sensu stricto—B31, isolated from a tick and 297, isolated from cerebrospinal fluid of a patient with neuroborreliosis.

Four different peptide ELISA tests were developed based on IR6 regions of two *B. burgdorferi* sensu stricto strains (B31 and 297), of one *B. afzelii* (PT7) and one *B. garinii* (IP90) strain. Two different serum panels were tested. The first one consisted of serum samples from Bulgarian patients with Lyme borreliosis—50 sera from patients with erythema migrans (clinical hallmark of early Lyme borreliosis), 20 sera from patients with neuroborreliosis, and 10 sera from patients with Lyme arthritis. This serum panel was used to analyze sensitivity of the tests. It contained 40 serum samples from patients with known cross-reactive serological results—patients with syphilis (n = 10), leptospirosis (n = 10), rheumatoid arthritis (n = 10), and sclerodermia (n = 10). The second serum panel was applied to test specificity of the developed peptide ELISA tests.

Test results showed that the two C6 peptides from *B. burgdorferi* sensu stricto had higher reactivity than the corresponding C6 peptides from *B. afzelii* and *B. garinii* with sera from patients with erythema migrans and those with Lyme arthritis. On the contrary, the C6 peptide from *B. garinii* was more reactive with sera from patients with neuroborreliosis [3]. The two peptides from *B. burgdorferi* sensu stricto showed different reactivity with sera from patients with erythema migrans (**Table 1**).

Concerning non-specific reactivity of the peptide antigens with sera from patients with syphilis, leptospirosis, rheumatoid arthritis, and sclerodermia, the lowest level of specificity (87.5%) was found for the C6 peptide from *B. afzelii*; specificity was higher (90% and 92.5%) with the C6 peptides from *B. burgdorferi* s.s. and highest (100%) with the C6 from *B. garinii*. Overall, specificity of the four peptides was high [3].

In order to test applicability of the C6 peptide for serological diagnosis, we used peptide ELISA tests for detection of antibodies in Lyme borreliosis. Four peptide antigens from the C6 regions of VlsE proteins from the three *Borrelia* species that mainly cause Lyme disease in Europe were tested. The findings were very promising since up to 80% of the patients with early Lyme borreliosis and neuroborreliosis and all patients with Lyme arthritis can be diagnosed by the peptide ELISA tests. In addition, overall specificity of the C6 tests was high (87.5–100%). Notably, the tests are easy to perform and cheap as the peptide synthesis is much more easy to implement than the production of recombinant protein antigens.

The C6 peptides from *B. burgdorferi* sensu stricto showed the highest sensitivity in detection of specific anti-borrelia antibodies in patients with early Lyme disease

Serum panel	**C6 B31 (*B. burgdorferi* s.s.)**	**C6 297 (*B. burgdorferi* s.s.)**	**C6 IP90 (*B. garinii*)**	**C6 PT7 (*B. afzelii*)**
Erythema migrans (n = 50)	36 (72%)	39 (78%)	26 (52%)	29 (58%)
Neuroborreliosis (n = 20)	11 (55%)	11 (55%)	16 (80%)	9 (45%)
Lyme arthritis (n = 10)	10 (100%)	10 (100%)	8 (80%)	8 (80%)
Total number of reacted samples (% sensitivity)	57 (71.3%)	60 (75%)	50 (62.5%)	46 (57.5%)
Number of reactive sera from patients with other diseases (% specificity)	3/40 (92.5%)	4/40 (90%)	0 (100%)	5/40 (87.5%)

Table 1.
Reactivity of peptide C6 ELISA with serum panels of patients with Lyme disease in Bulgaria.

from Bulgaria. Our previous studies on borrelia infections of Bulgarian ticks have shown that the ticks are mostly infected with *B. afzelii*, followed *by B. burgdorferi* sensu stricto and *B. garinii* [4]. The discrepancy between the abundance of *B. afzelii* in our ticks and predominant *B. burgdorferi* sensu stricto reactivity of Lyme borreliosis patients could be explained by different pathogenic potential of the *Borrelia* species.

It is well known that different *Borrelia* species cause predominantly certain clinical manifestations: neuroborreliosis is associated with *B. garinii* and Lyme arthritis with *B. burgdorferi* sensu stricto [5]. This finding may explain the higher reactivity of sera from patients with neuroborreliosis with the C6 peptide from *B. garinii* as well as the predominant reactivity of the sera from Lyme arthritis with the C6 from *B. burgdorferi* sensu stricto.

1.4 PCR detection of *Borrelia*, *Ehrlichia*, and *Rickettsia* DNAs in *I. ricinus* ticks from Bulgaria

A total of 298 *I. ricinus* ticks, collected by flag from the vegetation in 2000 and 2001, were examined by the reverse line blotting technique for *Borrelia, Ehrlichia,* and *Rickettsia* DNAs [6].

Prevalence of *Borrelia*, *Ehrlichia*, and *Rickettsia* in 202 ticks, collected in 2000, was as follows. Overall *Borrelia* prevalence in adult ticks was 41% (44% in males and 39% in females) and 10% in nymphs. *B. afzelii* was the predominant species. Its prevalence was 23% (26 of 112) in adult ticks and 6% (5 of 90) in nymphs, representing 56% (31/55) of all *Borrelia*-positive results. *B. burgdorferi* sensu stricto was detected in 15 (13%) of 112 adult ticks and in 1 (1%) of 90 nymphs. Prevalence of *B. garinii* was 3% in adult ticks and 7% in nymphs. *B. valaisiana* was detected in 3 and *B. lusitaniae* in other 3 of 202 examined ticks.

Overall *Borrelia* prevalence in adult *I. ricinus* ticks, collected in 2001, was 29% (21 of 72) in adult ticks (8% in males and 40% in females). No *Borrelia* infection was found in nymphs from 2001. *B. afzelii* was again the prevalent species—prevalence rate 15% (11 of 72) in adult ticks, representing 52% (11/21) of all *Borrelia*-positive results. Prevalences of *B. garinii* and *B. valaisiana* were 7% and 8%, respectively.

Anaplasma phagocytophilum was detected in 36 (32%) of 112 adult ticks and in 5 (6%) of 90 nymphs, collected in 2000. Of the ticks, collected in 2001, *A. phagocytophilum* was detected in 28% of adult ticks (male 17% and female 33%) and 21% of nymphs.

Of 202 *I. ricinus* ticks, collected in 2000, 94 (47%) were found to carry *Rickettsia* DNA: 78% of males, 61% of females, and 19% of nymphs. Prevalence of *R. helvetica* was 28% (56/202) and prevalence of IRS4 rickettsia was 30% (60/202). *R. conorii* was found in only two of the ticks. Ticks, collected in 2001, showed also high *Rickettsia* infectivity rate, 40% (38 of 96): 83% in males, 29% in females, and 17% in nymphs. *R. helvetica* was again the prevalent species, detected in 18% and 23% of the ticks, respectively.

A high proportion of Bulgarian *I. ricinus* ticks contains *Borrelia* DNA. Analysis of *Borrelia* prevalence revealed that ticks, collected from the same location and even in the same month (May) but in 2 adjacent years, 2000 and 2001, had different *Borrelia* prevalence (41% and 29%, respectively). Apart differences in overall *Borrelia* prevalence, there were also differences in *Borrelia* prevalence in males, females, and nymphs, collected in the 2 years in the same place. In ticks from 2000, *Borrelia* was most prevalent in adult males, less so in adult females and least so in nymphs, while in ticks from 2001, the prevalence was higher in females and lower in males and nymphs.

B. afzelii is highly prevalent among Bulgarian *I. ricinus* ticks, giving more than half of the *Borrelia*-positive results, followed by *B. burgdorferi* sensu stricto, *B. garinii, B. valaisiana*, and *B. lusitaniae* in that order. Prevalence of coinfection is high (17–45%) in *Ixodes* ticks, representing double or even triple infection with *Borrelia*, *Ehrlichia*, and/or *Rickettsia*. Even coinfection with two different *Borrelia* or *Ehrlichia* species was often detected, showing that the tick hosts are infected with multiple tick-borne pathogens. Since these ticks were collected from vegetation, a risk for simultaneous transmission of these pathogens during the same tick bite exists.

2. Crimean-Congo hemorrhagic fever

2.1 Introduction

Crimean-Congo hemorrhagic fever (CCHF) is a tick-borne human viral disease with a fatality rate up to 30%. It is characterized by a sudden onset of fever and muscular pain, often progressing to hemorrhagic manifestations [7]. Various wild and domestic mammals are natural reservoir hosts of CCHF virus (CCHFV). Ticks of the genus *Hyalomma* are primary vector and serve also as reservoir hosts. *Rhipicephalus* and *Dermacentor* ticks may play an additional role in maintaining the circulation of CCHFV in an enzootic cycle between vertebrates and ticks. The vector-competent ticks stay infected through the molt ("transovarial transmission") [7]. Humans are infected by infected ticks and also by contact with tissues or body fluids of infected animals or patients. Nosocomial outbreaks are described [8]. A case of probable airborne transmission is reported [9].

CCHF is spread in over 50 countries in Africa, Southern Asia, the Middle East, and Southeastern Europe, including the Balkan Peninsula. Cases have been reported in Bulgaria, Turkey, Kosovo, Albania, and Greece. CCHFV (genus *Orthonairovirus*, family *Nairoviridae*) is a negative-stranded RNA virus with a three-segmented genome: large (L), medium (M), and small (S) segments. CCHFV strains belong to seven genetic lineages. Lineage V, also named Europe 1, contains pathogenic CCHFV strains. Lineage VI, called Europe 2, contains genetically different Greek AP92 strains and recently reported similar strains from Turkey, Greece, Kosovo, and Algeria. Besides the detection in ticks, CCHFV lineage Europe 2 has been detected in a mild CCHF case in Turkey [10]. A fatal case due to an AP92-like strain has been recently reported in Iran [11].

With sporadic cases or small outbreaks, CCHF appeared in Bulgaria every year since 1950s. CCHFV was first detected in 1952 in Stara Zagora region [12]. Over 1500 cases have been reported in the country since then. For the last 10 years, 2009–2018, a total of 60 CCHF cases are officially recorded in the country. Case fatality rate of CCHF was an average 15.0%. There is a tendency for CCHF to spread in previously non-endemic areas. The strains causing CCHF in the country are closely related to others in the Balkan peninsula, belonging to lineage Europe 1 [13].

2.2 Countrywide seroprevalence study on Crimean-Congo hemorrhagic fever in general population of Bulgaria

To test current circulation of CCHFV in the country, we conducted a seroepidemiological study. The main objective of the study was to estimate the prevalence of IgG antibodies to CCHFV, as stable and long-persisting antibodies, in general human population of Bulgaria.

Serum samples were collected prospectively from 1500 residents of all 28 districts in Bulgaria. Participants were selected randomly among persons referred to public biochemistry laboratories in the regional primary healthcare centers to follow noninfectious diseases or for routine prophylactic checkup. Persons previously vaccinated against CCHFV were excluded from the study.

All serum samples were tested for anti-CCHFV IgG antibodies using commercially available ELISA kits according to the manufacturer's instructions (Vector-Best, Novosibirsk, Russia). Positive serum samples were tested also for specific IgM antibodies against CCHFV by ELISA kits from the same manufacturer. Positive samples for CCHFV IgG antibodies were additionally tested by commercial immunofluorescent kits (Euroimmun, Lübeck, Germany).

Specific IgG antibodies to CCHFV were found in 55 (3.7%) of the 1500 people tested by both ELISA and IFA tests. No CCHFV IgM antibodies were detected in these 55 samples. Analysis of the risk factors revealed that age over 40 years, tick bites, contact with livestock and residency in Haskovo district, are associated (95% CI) with an increased risk of CCHF [14].

Positive samples were found in residents of 20 out of the 28 districts in Bulgaria (**Figure 1**). The highest seroprevalence rate was observed in Southeastern Bulgaria: in districts of Haskovo (28%) and Yambol (12%), both well-known endemic regions. Notably, considerable seroprevalence rates were detected in districts where no CCHF cases have been reported, like in some northern and western districts [14].

A few CCHF cases are reported every year in Bulgaria. Nevertheless, results of the seroprevalence study revealed that actual significance of the disease is much higher with a high rate of subclinical infections. The mean established CCHF seroprevalence is comparable to those in other Balkan countries: 4.2% in Greece [15] and 4.0% in Kosovo [16]. The seroprevalence in the endemic Bulgarian districts is close to that in the endemic Turkish regions [17, 18], experiencing a large outbreak.

As found in previous studies, risk factors for CCHFV seropositivity are contact with livestock and tick bites. At higher risk are also residents of Haskovo district, where the highest seroprevalence is detected. There is no significant difference between the age groups. Nevertheless, there is significant difference in the

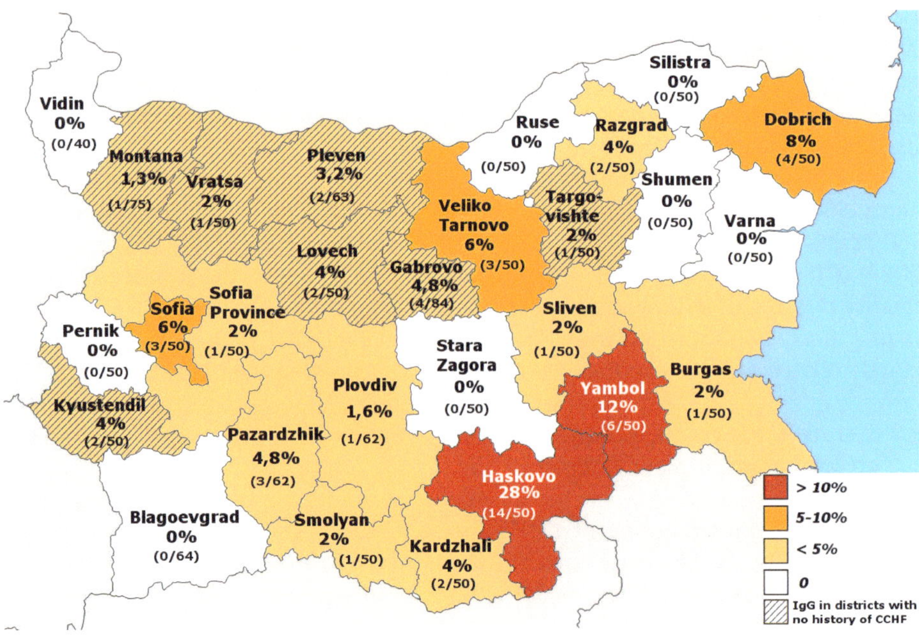

Figure 1.
CCHF seroprevalence by districts in Bulgaria.

seroprevalence rates in groups over and bellow 40 years. However, probability of contacting the virus also increases with age.

In the last years, almost all CCHF cases in Bulgaria are reported in southeastern districts, close to the national borders with Greece and Turkey (districts of Kardzhali, Yambol, Haskovo, and Burgas). On the other side, specific IgG antibodies against CCHFV were found in almost all Bulgarian districts (in 20 of 28 districts), high seroprevalence in the endemic districts, located in Southeastern Bulgaria, Haskovo (28%) and Yambol (12%), and significant seroprevalence in non-endemic areas in Northern and Western Bulgaria. The data presented indicate two important findings: (1) CCHFV increased substantially its circulation in the endemic regions and (2) CCHFV was introduced in many new areas.

In addition, the seroprevalence data revealed that CCHF may go asymptomatic or present with very mild manifestation in many cases. Increased awareness among physicians about subclinical forms of CCHF is needed.

2.3 Crimean-Congo hemorrhagic fever virus lineages Europe 1 and Europe 2 in Bulgarian ticks

In order to determine prevalence of CCHFV in ticks, a total of 2315 ixodid ticks were collected from 216 animals (cattle and sheep) in five Bulgarian districts, where CCHF cases were reported in the last 5 years, namely, Blagoevgrad, Kardzhali, Haskovo, Yambol, and Burgas. The majority of the ticks (2231/2315) were adults and the rest (84/2315) were nymphs.

By real-time reverse transcription polymerase chain reaction (RT-PCR), 623 *H. marginatum* and 107 *R. sanguineus* s.l. ticks were examined [19]. CCHFV RNA was detected in none of *R. sanguineus* s.l. ticks and in 39 of *H. marginatum* ticks (6.3%). The CCHFV RNA-positive ticks were collected from 13 animals: 9 cattle and 4 sheep (6% of all 216 domestic animals tested) in the districts of Burgas and Kardzhali, where the mean percentage of infected animals was 10.0% and 11.4%, respectively. (range 3.7%–17.7%). All positive samples were further tested by the RT-nested PCR. A total of 28 (71.8%) of them were again positive. Sequencing of these samples showed that they clustered into CCHFV lineage Europe 1. Average 8.8% of investigated *H. marginatum* ticks in Burgas and 8.6% in Kardzhali districts were infected with CCHFV. Infestation rate ranged per village from 2.7 to 15.2% [20].

Specific RT-nested PCR for CCHFV lineage Europe 2 [10] was applied to test negative real-time RT-PCR *R. sanguineus* s.l. ticks. A total of 49 (11.8%) of 415 investigated *R. sanguineus* s.l. ticks were positive. Very high rate of AP92-like CCHFV was found in *R. sanguineus* s.l. ticks from Kardzhali district (40.4%). In the district of Haskovo, infestation rate was 2.6%. Europe 2 lineage CCHFV was not detected in districts of Blagoevgrad, Burgas, and Yambol (**Figure 2**). Sequences were submitted to the GenBank DataBase (accession numbers KR092373, KR092374, and KX227372-KX227377) [20].

Detection of CCHFV lineage Europe 1 only in *H. marginatum* ticks supports its leading role as competent vector for CCHFV in Bulgaria. It is of interest that *H. marginatum* tick species is the predominant species in the two CCHF endemic districts: Kardzhali and Burgas. In some villages in these districts, *H. marginatum* ticks were infected with CCHFV up to 13.9 and 15.2%, respectively. In other Balkan countries, rates of CCHFV infection in *H. marginatum* ticks are as follows: 9.1–10.9% in Turkey [21, 22] and 11–15% in Kosovo [23, 24], although in another study in Kosovo, CCHFV was not detected in ticks collected from livestock in otherwise highly endemic regions [16].

CCHFV lineage Europe 2 was detected for the first time in Bulgaria: in 40% (46/114) of ticks in Kardzhali district. The previous study showed that the seroprevalence in human population in Kardzhali and Burgas districts is also high [25].

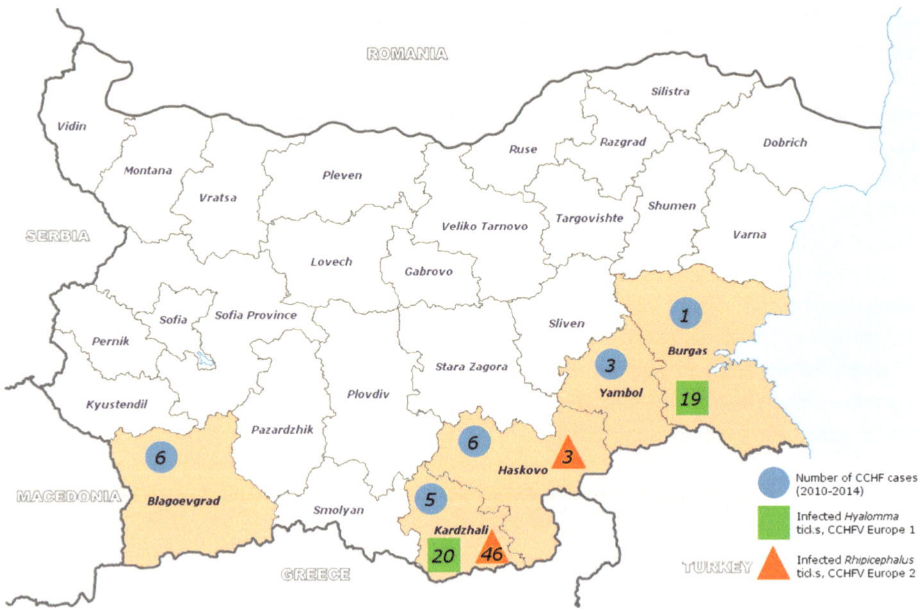

Figure 2.
Detection of CCHF virus lineages Europe 1 and Europe 2 in tick from Bulgaria.

Since CCHFV strain of lineage Europe 2 has been related with mild human disease in Turkey, the high infection rate of ticks in Kardzhali and Burgas districts may be connected with possible undetected mild or asymptomatic CCHF cases in these regions.

Summarizing the data, CCHFV lineages Europe 1 and Europe 2 were found in the district of Kardzhali. Both lineages were never detected simultaneously in ticks from an individual animal. One possible explanation could be superinfection exclusion of closely related viruses. All sequences from *R. sanguineus* s.l. ticks belong to CCHFV Europe 2 lineage. This lineage has been originally detected in *R. bursa* ticks from Greece, and much later similar sequences were detected in *R. bursa* and *H. marginatum* ticks in Turkey, in *R. bursa* ticks in Kosovo, in *H. aegyptium* ticks in Algeria, as well in a fatal CCHF case in Iran.

The tick study showed that Bulgarian ticks are infected at higher rate with the low pathogenic CCHFV lineage Europe 2 than with the high pathogenic lineage Europe 1 [20]. Possible widespread circulation of the low pathogenic CCHFV lineage Europe 2 strains might explain the discrepancy between high seroprevalence rates in humans and only few CCHF cases detected per year.

Further studies are needed especially where Europe 2 CCHFV strains were detected in order to investigate any association with human disease. In the area where Europe 1 lineage was detected, increased awareness about its pathogenicity to humans is needed.

3. Tick-borne encephalitis

3.1 Introduction

Tick-borne encephalitis is the most common tick-borne viral infection in humans. The disease occurs in North and Central Europe, Russia, Far East Asia, and Japan. In the last few decades, the number of reported cases increased within the endemic regions along with expanding of these areas.

Tick-borne encephalitis virus (TBEV) belongs to genus *Flavivirus*, family *Flaviviridae* like etiological agents of dengue, yellow fever, Zika infection, West Nile fever (WNF), and Japanese encephalitis. Three subtypes of the virus, European, Siberian, and Far Eastern, cause TBE with different severity and outcome of the disease.

Transmission routes of TBEV include bites of infected *Ixodes ricinus* ticks and consumption of row milk from infected goats, sheep, and cows. The incubation period is usually 7–14 days (between 2 and 28 days).

Like infections with other flaviviruses, most of the human infections with TBEV are asymptomatic (75–98%). Among the symptomatic patients infected with European subtype of TBEV, most develop unspecific febrile disease. In some cases only, infection of the central nervous system appears—meningitis (about 50% of the patients), meningoencephalitis (about 40%), and meningoencephalomyelitis (about 10%).

Tick-borne encephalitis is very unusual in Bulgaria. Over the past 40 years, only a few cases of TBE have been detected. Most of the TBE cases in the country are due to consumption of row goat milk. However, the tick vector, *Ixodes ricinus*, is widely distributed in Bulgaria, and Lyme borreliosis, transmitted by the same tick species, is endemic in the country.

Since 2009, reliable laboratory diagnosis of TBE, based on PCR and ELISA, was introduced, and the first three confirmed TBE cases in Bulgaria were identified: two cases in 2009 and one case in 2012 [26]. Two more TBE cases are identified in 2015.

3.2 A nationwide seroprevalence screening for tick-borne encephalitis virus in the population of Bulgaria

To assess local circulation and risk for human infections with TBEV, nationwide seroprevalence study was conducted in 2015 for the first time in Bulgaria.

Serum samples were prospectively collected from persons visiting laboratories for routine checkup in primary healthcare centers in all districts of Bulgaria: Blagoevgrad (n = 64), Gabrovo (n = 63), Vidin (n = 40), Montana (n = 78), Dobrich (n = 52), Plovdiv (n = 62), Targovishte (n = 42), and 50 samples from each of the rest 21 districts. Information about age, sex, and area of residence for each sampled person was collected in the laboratories.

Using ELISA kits (Euroimmun, Lübeck, Germany), all serum samples were tested for TBEV IgG antibodies. Then, all IgG-positive samples were tested for specific IgM antibodies by ELISA. In addition, avidity tests (from the same manufacturer) were applied to distinguish between acute and non-acute TBEV infections.

A total of 1451 residents of all districts in Bulgaria (population 7.2 million), 622 male and 829 female, the mean age ± standard deviation was 53.2 ± 18.8 years, were tested for TBEV-specific IgG antibodies.

Nine persons were found reactive by IgG ELISA; mean seroprevalence was 0.6%. IgM antibodies were not detected. IgG avidity index ranged from *33–85%*, main 60%. The nine people were residents of six districts. The highest seroprevalence rate was found in districts of Gabrovo (4.8%) and Ruse (4%) (**Figure 3**). No significant association between age and TBEV infection was detected [27].

The first and nationwide seroprevalence survey on TBEV circulation in Bulgaria found overall seroprevalence of 0.6% for TBEV. However, district analysis showed TBEV seroprevalence up to 4–4.8%. The great variability of IgG avidity indices is suggestive of recent and past infections.

TBE is endemic in Central and Northern European countries. By occasion, TBE has been detected in Southern Europe and the Balkan Peninsula in particular. Nevertheless, data obtained from the seroprevalence study indicates noticeable appearance of TBEV infections in Bulgaria.

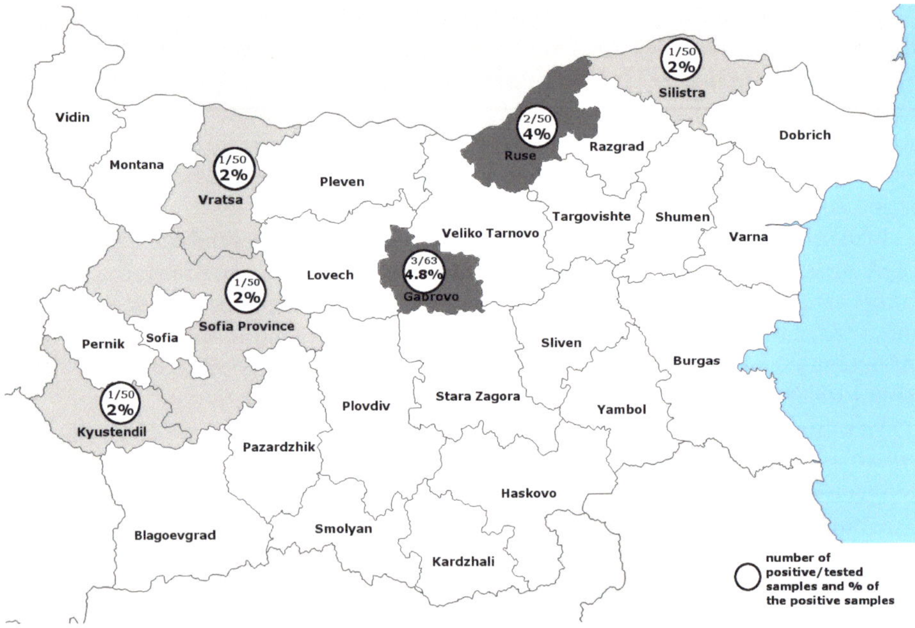

Figure 3.
TBEV seroprevalence in Bulgaria, 2015.

The level of TBEV seroprevalence in Bulgaria showed that the infection seems to be more widespread in the country as has been described so far. It is evidence that some viral encephalitis or meningoencephalitis cases in the country are underdiagnosed and underreported.

3.3 Tick-borne encephalitis among patients with viral meningitis in Bulgaria

Considering the remarkable increase in TBE morbidity in Europe over the past two decades [28], we organized and conducted a study of TBE among patients with acute viral meningitis, who were hospitalized in Bulgaria during 2009–2012.

A total of 86 patients with acute viral meningitis were investigated between 2009 and 2012 by physicians at the infectious diseases units at regional hospitals in districts of Sofia, Pazardzhik, Plovdiv, and Burgas. A total of 86 serum samples were collected during the acute phase and 49 sera at the convalescence phase up to 30 days after the first sample.

All 135 serum samples from patients were tested for IgM antibodies, and positive were also tested for IgG antibodies against TBE virus using commercially available ELISA tests (Euroimmun, Germany), according to the manufacturer's instructions.

TBE virus RNA was detected by reverse transcription polymerase chain reaction based on quantitative real-time technology (TaqMan) as described [29]. The system detected a fragment of the 3′ noncoding region of the TBE virus genome.

A total of 86 patients with viral meningitis of unknown etiology during this period were tested to detect acute TBE. Three TBE cases in Bulgaria were found. The last TBE case was detected in October 2012 and the other two were diagnosed in 2009.

3.3.1 Case no. 1

A girl aged 16 years residing in Velingrad (South Bulgaria) was admitted to the regional hospital on April 10, 2009. The patient had a high fever (40°C) and malaise. The temperature went to normal 3–4 days after admission, and then again her condition deteriorated with fever, headache, stiff neck, sore throat, nausea, vomiting, and depressed mood. The patient had a history spending some time in the forest. The cerebrospinal fluid (CSF) collected on April 14 showed a high number of leucocytes (160/μL; norm, 0–5/μL) with 75% granulocytes, high protein content (125 mg/dL, norm 15–45 mg/dL), and normal glucose level (0.31 mmol/L; norm, 0.22–0.44 mmol/L). The patient was transferred to a hospital in Sofia and a second CSF sample was obtained on April 22, 2009. The CSF flow was at increased pressure, leucocytes count was 400/μL (norm: 0–5/μL) with 65% lymphocytes, the protein content was 100 mg/dL (norm 15–45 mg/dL), and glucose level was normal. *Mycobacterium tuberculosis* was isolated from this CSF sample. TBE virus was detected by real-time RT-PCR [29] in the serum sample drawn on April 14. The serum sample drawn on April 22 showed high titers of specific IgM antibodies against TBE virus by enzyme-linked immunosorbent assay (ELISA) (Euroimmun, Germany). IgG antibodies against TBE virus were not found.

3.3.2 Case no. 2

On September 11, 2009, a 21-year-old man was admitted to the regional hospital in Plovdiv (South Bulgaria) with fever (38.5°C), fatigue, headache, nausea, and vomiting. Stiff neck, stupor, muscle soreness, conjunctivitis, and abnormal reflexes with pain in joints were found during physical examination. The onset of the disease was 5–6 days earlier. Exposure to tick bites could be excluded. The CSF analysis showed increased count of leucocytes 301/μL (norm: 0–5/μL) with 82% lymphocytes, slightly elevated protein (56 mg/dL; norm, 15–45 mg/dL), and normal glucose level (0.38 mmol/L; norm, 0.22–0.44 mmol/L). The patient initially improved and after a week, the patient's condition worsened again. He manifested fever, significant dizziness, and severe headache. The CSF analysis also supported worsening of the patient. Leucocyte count reached 442/μL (norm: 0–5/μL), with 90% lymphocytes, and protein was remarkably elevated (134 mg/dL; norm, 15–45 mg/dL); glucose level (0.28 mmol/L, norm, 0.22–0.44 mmol/L) was normal. Within a month, the patient gradually recovered. Examination by ELISA of paired serum samples from the patient, one upon admission and a second during the reconvalescence, revealed high level of IgM antibodies and no IgG antibodies in the first serum sample and borderline level of IgM antibodies in the first sample and significant levels of IgG antibodies against TBEV in the second serum sample [26].

3.3.3 Case no. 3

A 28-year-old woman, resident of Burgas area (East Bulgaria), was admitted to the regional hospital on September 23, 2012, with fever (37.5–38^0 C), significant numbness in muscles, and weakness. Physical examination revealed mild neck stiffness, mild left hemiparesis, and distal-type hypoesthesia. Her medical history started 2 days before. Upon admission, a tick was found on her body and removed. On September 27 the patient's condition improved, but starting from October 1, the fever, weakness, and numbness in muscles exacerbated. CSF analysis showed slightly elevated leukocytes (60/μL; norm, 0–5/μL) and protein (74 mg/dL; norm, 15–45 mg/dL), normal glucose level (0.38 mmol/L; norm, 0.22–0.44 mmol/L). Two serum samples, taken on October 1 and October 10 were tested by ELISA, and both antibodies, IgM and IgG, specific to TBE virus were detected. The patient was discharged in improved condition.

The serum samples of the three patients tested negative by ELISA and IFA for West Nile and yellow fever viruses, also negative for IgM antibodies to *Borrelia burgdorferi* by ELISA. Their CSF samples tested negative for bacterial culture. Though TBE cases are reported sporadically, TBE virus circulates in the country, causing human cases associated either with tick bites or consumption of unpasteurized milk.

In all three patients described, typical biphasic course of TBE infection was revealed. About two-thirds of the patients develop only febrile syndrome in the first phase of the disease [30]. Neurological disorders appear during the second febrile phase. Biphasic febrile illness is typical for infection with Western subtype of the virus. Patients infected with Eastern subtype of TBEV develop only monophasic course [30].

TBE cases in humans are occasionally reported in Bulgaria. However, the fact that TBE cases occur in Bulgaria, even sporadically, and are associated with tick bites or consumption of unpasteurized milk shows that TBE virus circulates in the country. Taking into account that patients who develop neurological symptoms are only "the tip of the iceberg"; one can predict that the real amount of infected people is many times more.

There is significant increase in the number of registered cases of TBE in Europe, Russia, and Far East, starting with 1990 [28]. Since then, about 10,000–12,000 TBE cases are reported annually in Europe and Russia. There is a tendency to global increase in the number of cases and to expansion of areas at risk. In Sweden, a significant increase in TBE cases reported was recorded in the last decade [31]. New endemic areas in Switzerland were confirmed by detection of TBE virus RNA in field-collected ticks [32]. Since September 2012, considering the importance and spread of TBE in the European Union, European Commission included TBE in the list of communicable diseases covered by epidemiological surveillance in the member states [33].

The three cases reported considered the first clinically and laboratory confirmed cases in Bulgaria since. The first case proved to have mixed infection with *M. tuberculosis* that could promote the primary progressive course of the meningoencephalitis, as previously reported [34]. The second case showed clinical manifestation of subacute viral meningitis, while the third case presented as subacute encephalomyelitis.

Usually, IgM and IgG antibodies to TBEV are present by the time that central nervous system involvement manifests in the second stage of TBE. Nucleic acids of the TBEV are very rarely detected by PCR during the viremic stage of the disease [29]. Surprisingly, we detected TBE virus infection by RT-PCR in the first patient. Thus, we confirmed not only the case but also the real circulation of the virus in Southeast Europe, where no information is available so far. The first case described above was also remarkable by the two coinfections ongoing—TBE and tuberculosis, responsible for aggravation of the course of the illness.

The TBE cases described showed that the disease is probably not uncommon in Bulgaria. The risk of TBE is underestimated in Bulgaria because of the low awareness of medical doctors. TBE should be taken into consideration in patients with various manifestations of central nervous system infections in Bulgaria.

4. West Nile fever

4.1 Introduction

West Nile virus (WNV) is a member of the genus *Flavivirus* within the *Flaviviridae* family. Widespread *Culex* mosquitoes transmit WNV.

About 80% of human infections with WNV are asymptomatic [32]. Around 20% of infections with WNV present as febrile syndrome and less than 1% manifest as neuroinvasive disease such as encephalitis, meningitis, or polio-like paralysis [35].

First in 2015, a few probable WNV human cases appeared in Bulgaria. Then, one confirmed WNV neuroinvasive infection was described [36]. The causative strain belonged to WNV lineage 2, closely related to Greek strains that caused the largest outbreak of WNV in Europe 2010–2013 [37] and also close to the WNV that caused outbreak in Hungary in 2008, when the WNV lineage 2 emerged for the first time outside Africa [38].

4.2 A nationwide seroprevalence screening for West Nile virus in the population of Bulgaria

To assess local circulation and risk for human infections with WNV, a nationwide seroprevalence study was conducted.

Serum samples were collected prospectively from persons visiting laboratories for routine prophylactic checkup in all districts of Bulgaria: Blagoevgrad (n = 64), Gabrovo (n = 63), Vidin (n = 40), Dobrich (n = 52), Plovdiv (n = 62), Targovishte (n = 42), Montana (n = 78), and 50 samples from each of the rest 21 districts. Information on age, sex, and area of residence for each sampled person was recorded by the staff in the laboratories.

Using ELISA kits (Euroimmun, Lübeck, Germany), serum samples were tested for WNV IgG antibodies. IgG-positive samples were further tested for specific IgM antibodies and for IgG avidity using the tests from the same manufacturer. Microneutralization assay (MNTA) was used to test all IgG-positive samples to exclude infection with closely related Usutu virus (USUV).

Serum samples from 1451 residents of all districts in Bulgaria, 622 male and 829 female, mean age ± standard deviation 53.2 ± 18.8 years, were tested for WNV-specific IgG antibodies.

Specific WNV IgG antibodies were detected in 22 participants tested by ELISA giving mean seroprevalence rate of 1.5%. Neutralizing antibodies were found in 6 (27.3%) of the IgG-positive samples; titer of these antibodies ranged between 1:10 and 1:100. The MNTA-positive samples originated from four districts (**Figure 4**). IgM antibodies were detected in two of the IgG-positive samples, and one of them was also MNTA-positive (titer 1:100) with IgG avidity index 48%. IgG avidity index for the rest of the MNTA-positive samples was between 70 and 97%. IgG avidity index of all samples ranged between 14 and 97%, mean 59%. USUV was not found in any serum samples.

The highest seroprevalence rates of WNV IgG antibodies were detected in districts of Sofia Province and Vidin—10 and 7.5%, respectively, followed by districts of Ruse and Silistra—6% each (**Figure 4**). There was no significant association of WNV seroprevalence neither with gender or age [27].

The first and nationwide seroprevalence survey on WNV circulation in Bulgaria found overall seroprevalence of 1.5% for WNV. However, district analysis showed WNV seroprevalence up to 7.5–10%. Recent and past infections could be suspected in accordance with variability of the IgG avidity indices.

Analysis of the WNV seroprevalence rates in Bulgaria showed that they are lower than the rates in the endemic European countries (Greece, Northern Italy, and Southern France) [37, 39, 40]. Nevertheless, they showed that WNV is widespread in the country. The highest WNV seroprevalence rate was detected in Sofia Province, where the first confirmed neuroinvasive case was described in 2015 [36] and an additional case was confirmed in 2016. WNV IgM antibodies were detected in people only from this district, giving a certainty that it is a “hot spot,” and more cases from this area could be expected in the future. WNV antibodies were detected in almost all districts near the river Danube, the border of Bulgaria with Romania. WNV outbreaks in Romania in 1996–1997 and 2010 appeared in areas close to the Bulgarian border [41]. This area represents excellent conditions for mosquito reproduction. At high risk for attracting WNV infection, according to the seroprevalence data, are also people in some central districts along the big rivers Maritsa and Tundzha as well as in a southern district, close to the border with Greece. The

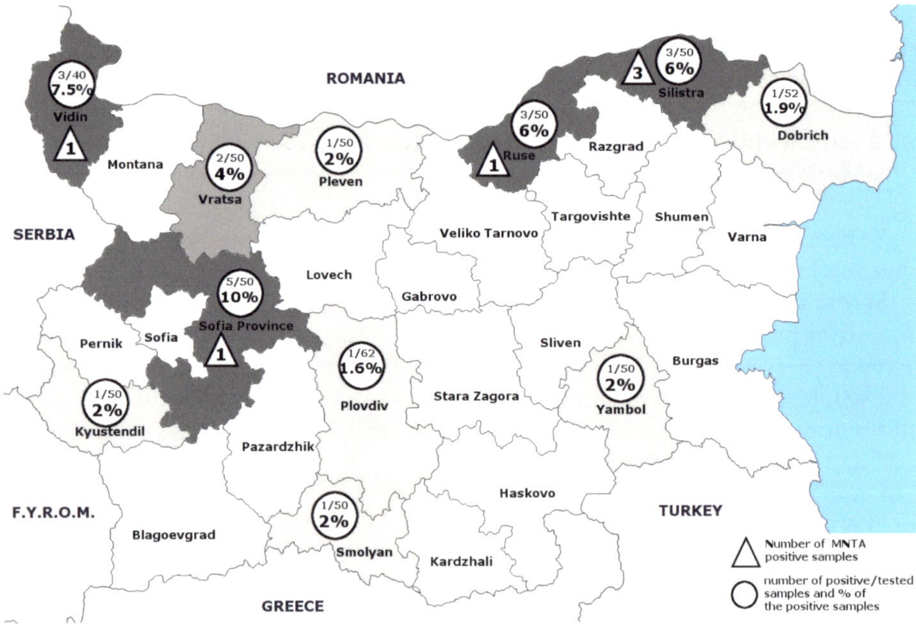

Figure 4.
WNV seroprevalence in Bulgaria, 2015.

big WNV outbreak in Greece, 2010–2012, affected northern parts of the country, not far from Bulgarian territory. The causative WNV was a recent introduction of WNV lineage 2 strain [42]. In the last years, WNV expanded and was reported also in other Balkan states.

WNF infection seems to be more widespread in the country as has been described so far. The level of WNV seroprevalence found in Bulgaria is evidence that some viral encephalitis or meningoencephalitis cases in the country are underdiagnosed and underreported.

Acknowledgements

This work has received funding from the European Union's Horizon 2020 research and innovation program under grant agreement No 732732.

Author details

Iva Christova
National Center of Infectious and Parasitic Diseases, Sofia, Bulgaria

*Address all correspondence to: iva_christova@yahoo.com

References

[1] Liang FT, Philipp MT. Epitope mapping of the immunodominant invariable region of *Borrelia burgdorferi* VlsE in three host species. Infection and Immunity. 2000;**68**:2349-2352

[2] McDowell JV, Sung S, Hu LT, Marconi RT. Evidence that the variable regions of the central domain of VlsE are antigenic during infection with Lyme disease spirochetes. Infection and Immunity. 2002;**70**:4196-4203

[3] Christova I, Trifonova I, Gladnishka T, Taseva E, Ivanova V, Rusimova D. C6 peptides from *Borrelia burgdorferi* sensu stricto, *Borrelia afzelii* and *Borrelia garinii* as antigens for serological diagnosis of Lyme borreliosis. Biotechnology & Biotechnological Equipment. 2014;**27**:3540-3542

[4] Christova I, Schous L, van De Pol I, Park J, Panayotov S, Lefterova V, et al. High prevalence of granulocytic Ehrlichiae and *Borrelia burgdorferi* sensu lato in *Ixodes ricinus* ticks from Bulgaria. Journal of Clinical Microbiology. 2002;**39**:4172-4174

[5] Balmelli T, Piffaretti JC. Association between different clinical manifestations of Lyme disease and different species of *Borrelia burgdorferi* sensu lato. Research in Microbiology. 1995;**146**:329-340

[6] Schouls L, van de Pol I, Rijpkema S, Schot C. Detection and identification of Ehrlichia, *Borrelia burgdorferi* sensu lato, and Bartonella species in Dutch *Ixodes ricinus* ticks. Journal of Clinical Microbiology. 1999;**37**:2215-2222

[7] Bente DA, Forrester NL, Watts DM, McAuley AJ, Whitehouse CA, Bray M. Crimean-Congo hemorrhagic fever: History, epidemiology, pathogenesis, clinical syndrome and genetic diversity. Antiviral Research. 2013;**100**:159-189

[8] Mardani M, Keshtkar-Jahromi M. Crimean–Congo hemorrhagic fever. Archives of Iranian Medicine. 2007;**10**:204-214

[9] Pshenichnaya NY, Nenadskaya SA. Probable Crimean-Congo hemorrhagic fever virus transmission occurred after aerosol-generating medical procedures in Russia: Nosocomial cluster. International Journal of Infectious Diseases. 2015;**33**:120-122

[10] Midilli K, Gargili A, Ergonul O, Elevli M, Ergin S, Turan N, et al. The first clinical case due to AP92 like strain of Crimean–Congo hemorrhagic fever virus and a field survey. BMC Infectious Diseases. 2009;**9**:90

[11] Salehi-Vaziri M, Baniasadi V, Jalali T, Mirghiasi SM, Azad-Manjiri S, Zarandi R, et al. The first fatal case of Crimean-Congo hemorrhagic fever due to AP92 like strain of Crimean-Congo hemorrhagic fever virus. Japanese Journal of Infectious Diseases. 2016;**69**:344-346

[12] Nekliudov M. A case of hemorrhagic fever (Crimean). Savremenna Med. 1952;**5**:92-95

[13] Papa A, Pappa S, Panayotova E, Papadopoulou E, Christova I. Molecular epidemiology of Crimean-Congo hemorrhagic fever in Bulgaria—An update. Journal of Medical Virology. 2016;**88**:769-773

[14] Christova I, Panayotova E, Trifonova I, Taseva E, Hristova T, Ivanova V. Country-wide seroprevalence studies on Crimean-Congo hemorrhagic fever and hantavirus infections in general population of Bulgaria. Journal of Medical Virology. 2017;**89**:1720-1725

[15] Sidira P, Maltezou HC, Haidich AB, Papa A. Seroepidemiological study of Crimean-Congo haemorrhagic

fever in Greece, 2009-2010. Clinical Microbiology and Infection. 2012;**18**:E16-E19

[16] Fajs L, Humoli I, Saksida A, Knap N, Jelovšek M, Korva M, et al. Prevalence of Crimean-Congo hemorrhagic fever virus in healthy population, livestock and ticks in Kosovo. PLoS One. 2014;**9**(11):e110982

[17] Koksal I, Yilmaz G, Aksoy F, Erensov S, Aydin H. The seroprevalence of Crimean-Congo hemorrhagic fever in people living in the same environment with Crimean-Congo hemorrhagic fever patients in an endemic region in Turkey. Epidemiology and Infection. 2014;**142**(2):239-245

[18] Ertugrul B, Kirdar S, Ersoy OS, Ture M, Erol N, Ozturk B, et al. The seroprevalence of Crimean-Congo hemorrhagic fever among inhabitants living in the endemic regions of western Anatolia. Scandinavian Journal of Infectious Diseases. 2012;**44**(4):276-281

[19] Garrison AR, Alakbarova S, Kulesh DA, Shezmukhamedova D, Khodjaev S, Endy TP, et al. Development of a TaqMan minor groove binding protein assay for the detection and quantification of Crimean–Congo hemorrhagic fever virus. The American Journal of Tropical Medicine and Hygiene. 2007;**77**:514-520

[20] Panayotova E, Papa A, Trifonova I, Christova I. Crimean-Congo hemorrhagic fever virus lineages Europe 1 and Europe 2 in Bulgarian ticks. Ticks and Tick Borne Diseases. 2016;**7**(5):1024-1028

[21] Ergönül O. Crimean-Congo haemorrhagic fever. The Lancet Infectious Diseases. 2006;**6**:203-214

[22] Yesilbag K, Aydin L, Dincer E, Alpay G, Girisgin AO, Tuncer P, et al. Tick survey and detection of Crimean–Congo hemorrhagic fever virus in tick species from a non-endemic area, South Marmara region, Turkey. Experimental and Applied Acarology. 2013;**60**:253-261

[23] Duh D, Saksida A, Petrovec M, Dedushaj I, Avsic-Zupanc T. Novel onestep real-time RT-PCR assay for rapid and specific diagnosis of Crimean–Congo hemorrhagic fever encountered in the Balkans. Journal of Virological Methods. 2006;**133**:175-179

[24] Sherifi K, Cadar D, Muji S, Robaj A, Ahmeti S, Jakupi X, et al. Crimean-Congo hemorrhagic fever virus clades V and VI (Europe 1 and 2) in ticks in Kosovo, 2012. PLoS Neglected Tropical Diseases. 2014;**8**:e3168

[25] Christova I, Gladnishka T, Taseva E, Kalvatchev N, Tsergouli K, Papa A. Seroprevalence of Crimean-Congo hemorrhagic fever virus, Bulgaria. Emerging Infectious Diseases. 2013;**19**:177-179. DOI: 10.3201/eid1901.120299

[26] Mohareb E, Christova I, Soliman A, Younan R, Kantardjiev T. Tick-borne encephalitis in Bulgaria, 2009-2012. Euro Surveillance. 2013;**18**(46)

[27] Christova I, Panayotova E, Tchakarova S, Taseva E, Trifonova I, Gladnishka T. A nationwide seroprevalence screening for West Nile virus and tick-borne encephalitis virus in the population of Bulgaria. Journal of Medical Virology. 2017;**89**(10):1875-1878

[28] Süss J. Tick-borne encephalitis in Europe and beyond—The epidemiological situation as of 2007. Euro Surveillance. 2008;**13**(26)

[29] Schwaiger M, Cassinotti P. Development of a quantitative real-time RT-PCR assay with internal control for the laboratory detection of tick borne encephalitis virus (TBEV) RNA. Journal of Clinical Virology. 2003;**27**:136-145

[30] Dumpis U, Crook D, Oksi J. Tick-borne encephalitis. Clinical Infectious Diseases. 1999;**28**(4):882-890

[31] Lundkvist A, Wallensten A, Vene S, Hjertqvist M. Tick-borne encephalitis increasing in Sweden. Euro Surveillance. 2011;**16**(39)

[32] Lommano E, Burri C, Maeder G, Guerne M, Bastic V, Patalas E, et al. Prevalence and genotyping of tick-borne encephalitis virus in questing *Ixodes ricinus* ticks in a new endemic area in western Switzerland. Journal of Medical Entomology. 2012;**49**(1):156-164

[33] European Commission decision. Official Journal of the European Union. L 239/3, 2012

[34] Meirova RA. Tick-borne encephalitis associated with other infections. Klin.Med. (Mosk). 1991;**69**(5):71-73

[35] Chancey C, Grinev A, Volkova E, Rios M. The global ecology and epidemiology of West Nile virus. BioMed Research International. 2015;**376230**. DOI: 10.1155/2015/376230

[36] Baymakova M, Trifonova I, Panayotova E, Dakova S, Pacenti M, Barzon L, et al. Fatal case of West Nile neuroinvasive disease in Bulgaria. Emerging Infectious Diseases. 2016;**22**(12):2203-2204. DOI: 10.3201/eid2212.151968

[37] Hadjichristodoulou C, Pournaras S, Mavrouli M, Marka A, Tserkezou P, Baka A, et al. West Nile virus seroprevalence in the Greek population in 2013: A Nationwide cross-sectional survey. PLoS One. 2015;**10**(11):e0143803. DOI: 10.1371/journal.pone.0143803

[38] Bakonyi T, Ivanics E, Erdelyi K, Ursu K, Ferenczi E, Weissenbock H, et al. Lineage 1 and 2 strains of encephalitic West Nile virus, Central Europe. Emerging Infectious Diseases. 2006;**12**:618-623

[39] Pierro A, Galbani P, Spadafora C, Ruggeri D, Randi V, Parenti S, et al. Detection of specific antibodies against West Nile and Usutu viruses in healthy blood donors in northern Italy, 2010-2011. Clinical Microbiology and Infection. 2013;**19**:E451-E453. DOI: 10.1111/1469-0691.12241

[40] Charrel R, de Lamballerie X, Durand JP, Gallian P, Attoui H, Biagini P, et al. Prevalence of antibody against West Nile virus in volunteer blood donors living in southeastern France. Transfusion. 2001;**41**:1-2

[41] Sirbu AC, Sirbu A, Celanu CS, Panculescu-Gatej R, Vazquez A, Tenorio A, et al. Outbreak of West Nile virus infection in humans. Euro Surveillance. 2010;**16**

[42] Dimou V, Gerou S, Papa A. The epidemic West Nile virus strain in Greece was a recent introduction. Vector Borne and Zoonotic Diseases. 2013;**13**(10):719-722

Section 4

Vector Control

Chapter 7

Use of Artificial Intelligence on the Control of Vector-Borne Diseases

Daniel da Silva Motta, Roberto Badaró, Alex Santos and Frank Kirchner

Abstract

Artificial intelligence has many fields of application with an increasing computational processing power, and the algorithms are reaching human performance on complex tasks. Entomological characterization of insects represents an essential activity to drive actions to control the vector-borne diseases. Identification of the species and sex of insects is essential to map and organize the control measurements by the public health system in most areas where transmission is actively occurring. In many places in the world, the methodology done for identification of the mosquitos is by visual examination from human trained researchers or technicians. This activity is time-consuming and requires several years of experience to have skills to do the job. This chapter addresses the application of artificial intelligence for identification of mosquitos associated with vector-borne diseases. Benefits, limitations, and challenges of the use of artificial intelligence on the control of vector-borne diseases are discussed in this review.

Keywords: artificial intelligence, machine learning, deep learning, mosquitoes classification, vector-borne diseases

1. Introduction

For those who are not familiar with artificial intelligence (AI), imagine that some tasks that are done by humans, such as object detection, visual interpretation, and speech recognition, can be done by computers without human interference. Why is that important? There are many benefits with the use of AI that we intend to discuss in this chapter.

AI is growing in fields that require algorithms (mathematical instructions for computers) and machines to solve problems that are intellectually difficult for human beings but relatively easy for programmable computers. Nevertheless, "the true challenge of AI is to solve tasks that are easy for people to perform, but hard to be described, once it requires intuition [1]." When we look at an image, our interpretation is instantaneous: Is there a car? Is there a person? Is there a house? Computers are able to interpret as well, but not in same way that humans do. Computers translate an image in numbers, as illustratively shown in **Figure 1**.

In the early years of artificial intelligence, a rapid growth has been experienced. "The AI index—2017 annual report, created at Stanford University, presents the volume of activities that involves AI. In this report, indicators help to understand the importance of artificial intelligence technologies for academia, industry, and

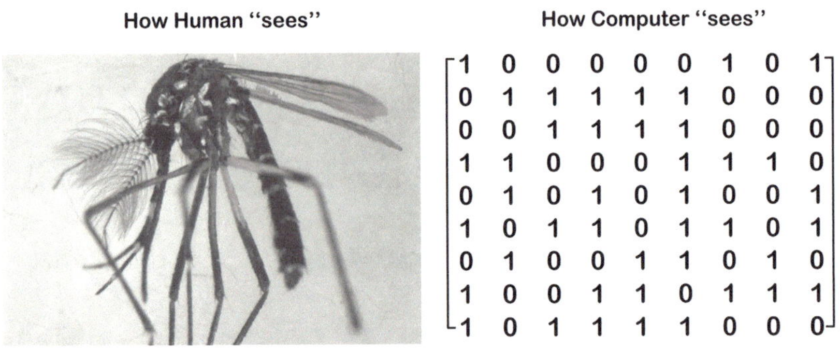

Figure 1.
Human vs. computer: how an image is recognized by each (illustrative).

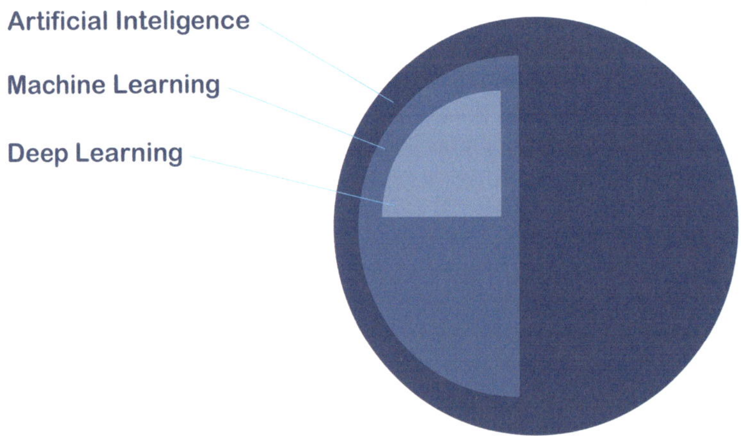

Figure 2.
Relationship between artificial intelligence, machine learning, and deep learning.

public sector. The number of AI published papers produced each year has increased by more than nine times since 1996. For industry, the number of active US startups developing AI systems has increased 14 times since 2000 [2]."

Machine learning (ML) is a subarea of artificial intelligence that is able to learn from previous experience. "ML algorithms are design to solve problems extracting features from existing data, learn from these features and predict the outcomes" [3]. For example, intelligent mosquito's trap can be designed with the functionality to classify harmful from beneficial insects, release the nontarget insects, and kill the target ones. The classifying process can previously learn from wingbeat frequency data of different species of insects, and whenever a new insect approaches the trap, it will automatically classify and take the decision—release it or kill it. That was exactly what "De Souza and Silva proposed using machine learning techniques" [4, 5].

Recently, "Deep Learning (DL) methods—a subarea of Machine Learning—are considered essential for general object recognition" [6]. "Tasks that consist of mapping an input to an output and that are easy for a person to do rapidly, can be accomplished via Deep Learning, given sufficiently large models and dataset of labeled training examples" [1]. "In the largest contest for object recognition, ImageNet Large Scale Visual Recognition Challenge (ILSVRC), a breakthrough for deep learning occurred in 2012 when a Deep Learning network won the competition, bringing the state-of-art top-5 error rate from 26.1% to 15.3%" [1]. **Figure 2** illustrates how artificial intelligence, machine learning, and deep learning are related.

An important field for application of artificial intelligence is health care. Based on the knowledge of medicine and historical data, AI can be used to support medical doctors to take better and faster decisions. For instance, AI can support medical doctors with robotics systems for some special tasks such as surgery, to increase the life expectancy of human beings, to increase the quality of life for people with some physical disability, and also to increase the community participation to improve the performance of a human care system.

In medicine, arboviruses have received a global attention, since "vector borne diseases are responsible for 17% of the estimated global burden of communicable diseases. It causes more than 700,000 deaths yearly and at least 80% of the global population lives in areas at risk" [7]. Entomology research is considered priority by the World Health Organization for the development of tools that can be applied to reduce incidence and mortality and prevent epidemics due to vector-borne diseases globally.

Identification of the species and sex of mosquitoes is essential to map and organize the control measurements by the public health system in most areas where transmission is actively occurring. In many places in the world, the methodology for identification of the mosquitos is done by visual examination from human trained technician. "This activity is time consuming and requires several years of experience to have skillful to do the job" [8].

This chapter addresses the application of artificial intelligence to help on the control of vector-borne diseases. Research trends and technologies connecting AI to vector-borne diseases are presented for a better understanding on how much researchers and institutions are becoming interested on both topics together. The use of machine learning and deep learning techniques, as a subarea of AI, is discussed for classification of mosquitos in their different life cycle—eggs, larval, pupal, and adult. Benefits and limitations are also presented to help the reader to understand the potential and challenges of artificial intelligence applied to entomology.

2. Research and technological trends on AI and vector-borne diseases

Since 2000, a continuous growth on published research (papers) and patents granted relating artificial intelligence with vector-borne diseases has been noticed. **Figure 3** represents the number of papers published yearly using the keywords: (insect OR mosquito OR culicid OR vector-borne OR zoonotic disease) AND (artificial intelligence OR machine learning OR deep learning). This review considered the following sources: IEEE, PlosOne, Capes, PubMed Web of Science, Current Contents Connect, Conference Proceedings, and Inspec.

It is interesting to notice that in 2017 the number of papers is almost six times it was in 2000. This result demonstrates that artificial intelligence has several possible applications on the control of vector-borne diseases as an important interest topic for many researchers around the world.

Figure 4 shows the number of patents granted in the world with the same keywords as the ones used for review papers. For the patents research, the platform Derwent Innovation was used.

In 2017, the number of patents granted is relevantly almost 10 times the average it was in the previous years. This result demonstrates that not only researchers but also companies have interest in intellectual property assets applying AI on the control of vector-borne diseases.

Figure 5 presents the top countries' and regions' intellectual properties' ownership. China, Korea, and Japan are the countries with more granted patents.

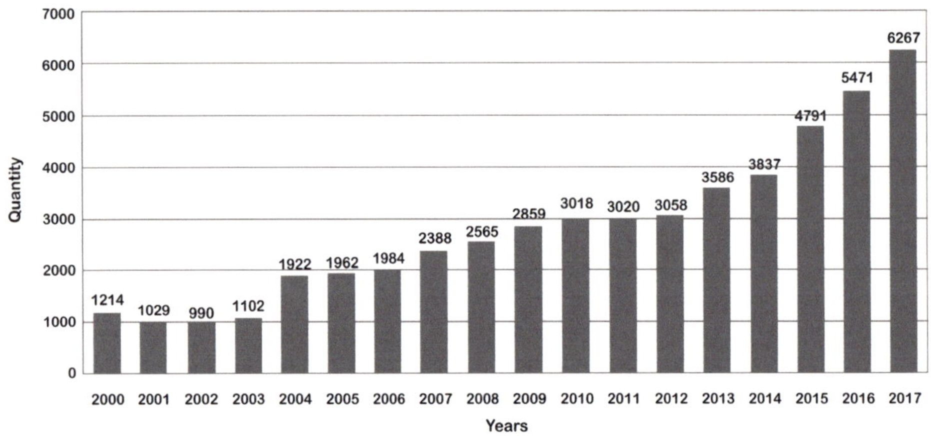

Figure 3.
The number of papers published from 2000 to 2017 relating AI to vector-borne diseases.

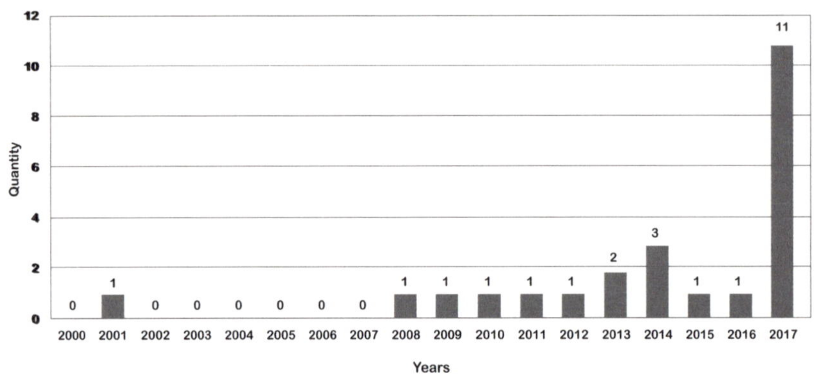

Figure 4.
The number of patents granted from 2000 to 2017 relating AI to vector-borne diseases.

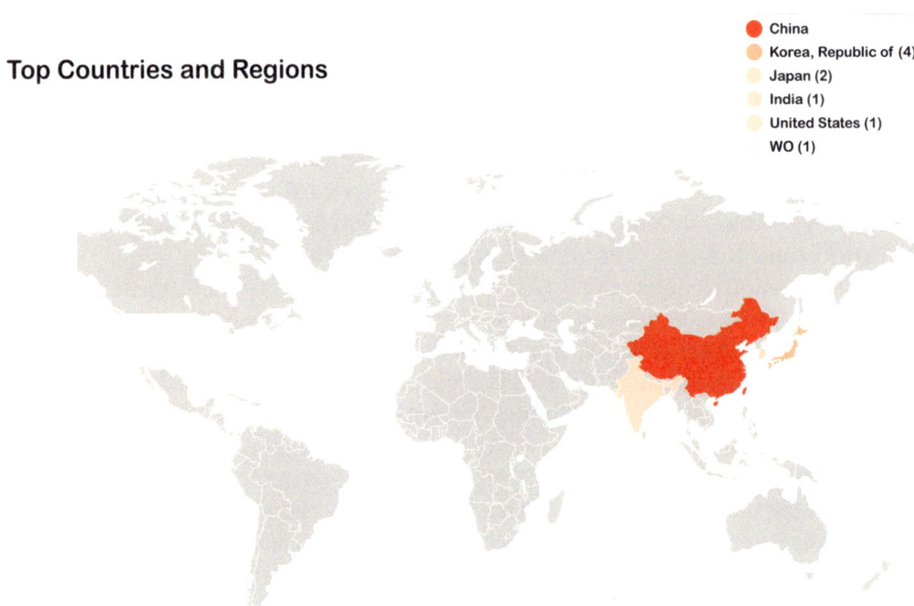

Figure 5.
Countries with more patents from 2000 to 2017 relating AI to vector-borne diseases.

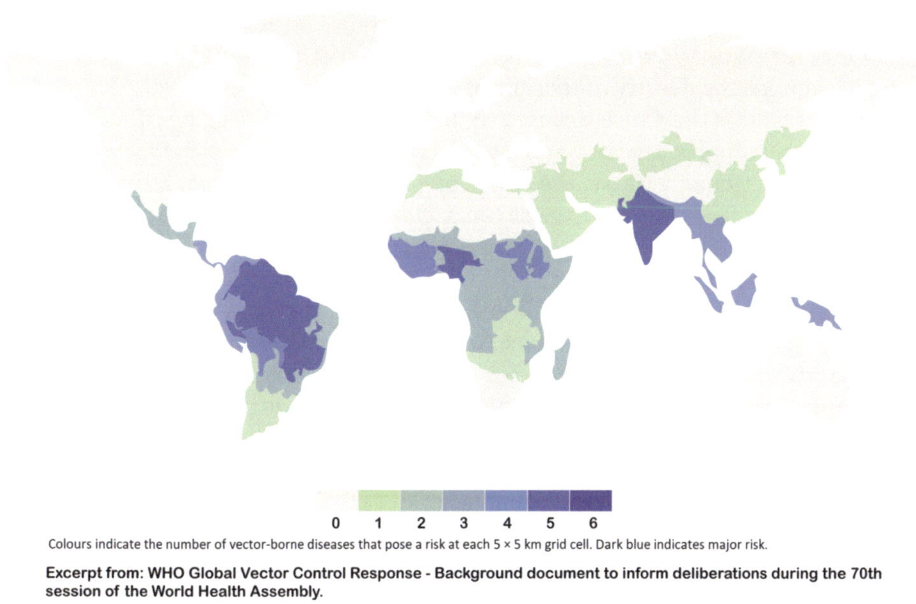

Figure 6.
Combined global distribution of seven major vector-borne diseases: malaria, lymphatic filariasis, leishmaniasis, dengue, Japanese encephalitis, yellow fever, and Chagas disease transmission [7].

Figure 6 presents the combined global distribution of seven major vector-borne diseases. Correlating **Figures** 5 and **6,** some countries that own IP relating AI to vector-borne diseases are not among the main ones that appear in "the global distribution of seven major vector-borne diseases for which integration of vector control programs may be beneficial—malaria, lymphatic filariasis, leishmaniasis, dengue, Japanese encephalitis, yellow fever and Chagas disease transmission—which evidences that vector borne is everyone's problem [7]."

3. How AI can benefit entomology

In this section, we present some benefits on applying artificial intelligence techniques in areas that are of high importance on the control of vector-borne diseases. Over the last year, much attention is being dedicated to capture and kill harmful mosquitoes using different kinds of mosquito's traps. Also, several methods have been developed to help mosquito's species classification process.

A major benefit on the application of AI is to increase the community participation in the control of vector-borne diseases and therefore successfully decrease the burden of arboviruses' recurrent epidemics.

3.1 Mosquito's trap

There are many mosquitos' traps available to capture and kill mosquitoes. Some of them are dedicated to attract females to deposit its eggs in the trap. Others are designed to capture and kill larva or adult mosquitoes.

Among the studies analyzed, some were dedicated to evaluate the performance of traps of capture of adult mosquitoes. "In [9], an approach is presented to remotely collect and identify field mosquitoes captured by two traps, "BG-trap" and "CDC light." The motivation of the work is justified considering that the activity of capture and classification requires the presence of entomological specialists and, therefore, faces constraints of budget and logistic feasibility."

Entomologists recognize that monitoring the traps is crucial to accomplishing its goal. Once the traps attract mosquito's female, if not periodically monitored, it might increase the density of mosquitos in the area the trap is located.

Another issue is the damage caused in the mosquito's body during the capture process. Some samples have its parts destroyed and also dried, what makes difficult the taxonomist's job to evaluate the morphological characteristics of the mosquito's species. **Figure 7** presents an image of *Culex quinquefasciatus* from Fiocruz—Oswaldo Cruz Foundation in Brazil. Some of the morphological characteristics are no longer presented in the sample.

Artificial intelligence can help the design of mosquito's traps by incorporating new important functions. For instance, it helps identify the targeted mosquitoes and separate from the nontargeted ones. Also, using AI, it is possible to acquire and store important information that can help to understand the mosquito's behavior and correlate data such as date and time of capture, species captured, and environmental data (humidity and temperature).

The application of machine learning techniques to design intelligent traps, using a laser sensor, and audio analysis techniques have been used to help insect recognition [5]. The device developed by the authors is able to attract and distinguish harmful from beneficial insects. Also let free the nontarget insects and kill the target ones, which can provide information to estimate the density of the target insect population. Different feature sets from audio analysis and machine learning algorithms achieved 98% accuracy in the insect classification.

Another example was the development of an automatic mosquito classification system consisted of an infrared recording device for profiling the wingbeat of the in-flight mosquito species. Also, a machine learning model was used for classifying the gender, genus, and species of the incoming mosquitoes by the signatures of their wingbeats [10]. To assess the performance of the system, the authors used living male and female *Aedes albopictus*, *Aedes aegypti*, and *Culex quinquefasciatus*. The results show that the accuracies of the proposed system are above 80% on identifying the gender and genus of the mosquitoes.

3.2 Mosquito classification

The correct identification of mosquito species is an essential step in the development of effective control strategies for vector-borne diseases. Ten years prior to

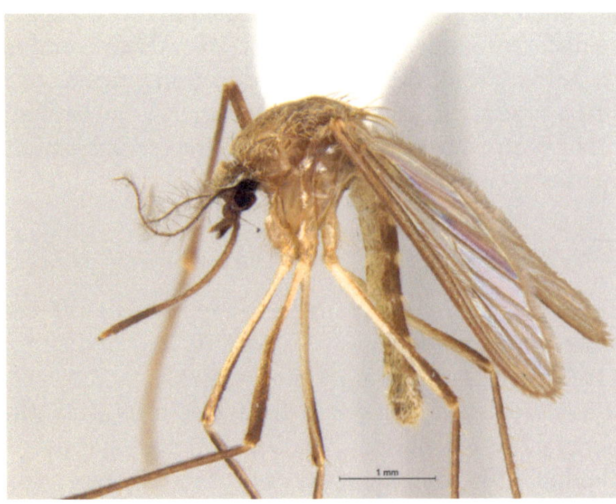

Figure 7.
Image of Culex quinquefasciatus from Fiocruz.

the occurrence of Zika virus, dengue, and chikungunya epidemic in Brazil, *Aedes aegypti* mosquito density increased almost 600 times.

Entomological characterization is fundamental to acquire information about mosquito's behavior. This activity requires trained and experienced personnel. "While the general interest in documenting species diversity has grown exponentially over the years, the number of taxonomists and other professionals trained in species identification has steadily declined [11, 12]."

According to Fiocruz, "the traditional method of classifying mosquitoes uses dichotomous keys [13]." These keys consist in analyzing morphological characteristics of the insect. "The dichotomous keys are mostly used to classify species beyond the 4th stage of larval phase" [14]. **Figure 8** represents the classification process using dichotomous keys for three different species—*Aedes aegypti*, *Aedes albopictus*, and *Culex quinquefasciatus*. The dichotomous keys are used to classify any species, not only the represented in **Figure 8** and uses images/figures/drawings to support the taxonomist during classification.

In order to use the dichotomous keys, the taxonomist needs to prepare the sample—if it is an adult, assemble the mosquito on entomological pin and observe the specimen under the microscope to evaluate the morphological characters. **Figure 9** represents the process of entomological characterization of an adult mosquito.

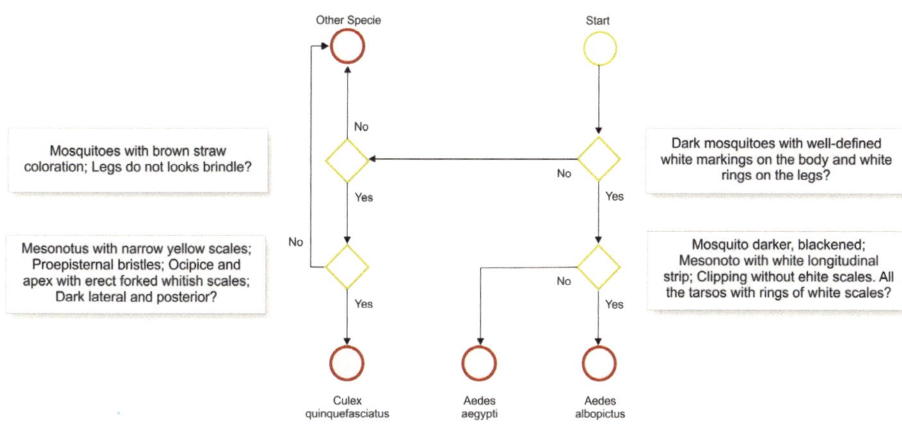

Figure 8.
Representation of the process using dichotomous keys for the classification of mosquitoes.

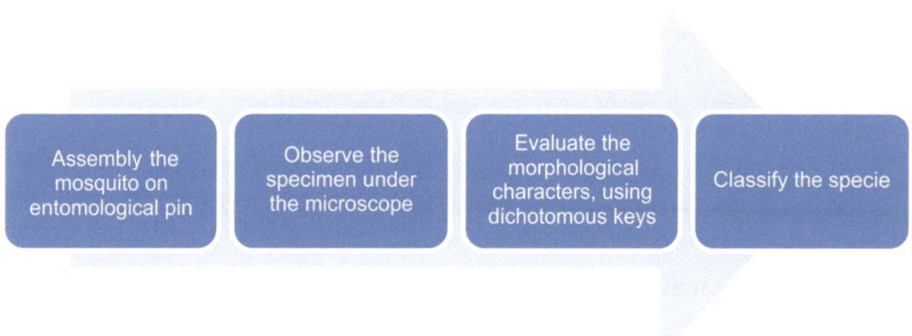

Figure 9.
Process of entomological characterization of an adult mosquito.

As already mentioned, some of the mosquito's samples are damaged and lose morphological characteristics during the capture in the field and the transport to a laboratory. Besides that, the waiting time during capture and transportation is also an issue and might dry the mosquito's body, which affect some characteristics such as color.

Another possibility for the "identification of species can be made through the use of molecular techniques that have been shown in different studies such DNA barcodes" [15]. Furthermore, molecular identification of mosquito remains a slow and expensive process for most laboratories.

Artificial intelligence can be applied to automatize the mosquito's classification process. It can be used to classify in field by entomologists or even nontaxonomists and health workers. By doing that, AI can avoid the major issues presented previously, like the need of trained and experienced personnel and lose of the morphological characteristics. Artificial intelligence application also allows increasing the number of mosquito's data, obtaining online information of population density, and the correlation with cases of incidence and mortality of vector-borne diseases.

In one AI application, deep learning was used to recognize *Aedes*-utilized wings morphology. "In [16], 17 species of the genera *Anopheles*, *Aedes*, and *Culex* were classified based on wing shape characteristics to test the hypothesis that classification using Artificial Intelligence was better than traditional classification method by discriminant analysis. The results demonstrated the AI correctly classified species more efficiently with an accuracy of 86%–100%."

Some authors study support vector machine (SVM) techniques. "In [17], the authors use digital image processing and support vector machine (SVM) to detect *Aedes aegypti* mosquito. It is suggested for a method of identification as binary key of mosquitoes from the visual identification of their morphology. A camera is integrated with a circuit board, where images are fed to a support vector machine, corresponding to body characteristics of the insect. Photos of insects are taken and then delivered to the machine for data comparison, where photo properties are valued and then matched. By the construction of the equipment, the system only responds if the identified mosquito is *Aedes aegypti* or not, to which it has an accuracy of 90% in the data."

In other applications, mosquito's larva digital images were used in a machine learning algorithm for *Aedes* larva identification. "The authors proposed a method to identify larvae of *Aedes* mosquitoes using convolutional neural networks (CNN), a new method in multilayer neural network technology that has proven its performance especially in image analysis. Larva's images were captured by cell phones. The classification method is divided into the following steps: 1) acquisition of images; 2) preprocessing the images; 3) CNN training; 4) Real-time classification. The results shown a good performance with 100% accuracy for identification of *Aedes* larva, however, for other mosquitoes the misclassification rate was 30% [18]." Although the sample size in this study was very small, it shows that artificial intelligence can be used for the mosquito's species classification.

4. Limitations and challenges on the application of ML and DL

Applications of machine learning and deep learning techniques in many areas are rapidly growing, due to the flexibility of their algorithms and also because it is not required to model previously the scenario using a mathematical function. Prototypes and computer systems are being developed, but there are still some bottlenecks to overcome. Although machine learning and deep learning algorithms are capable of capturing the complexity of several problems, in some cases the effective use of it depends on further research and development to increase the level of reliability before it can be used in the real world.

In this section, we present some limitation and challenges on the application of artificial intelligence, especially machine learning and deep learning techniques, which should be addressed in future researches.

4.1 Generic approach

An algorithm does not interpret a problem the same way that humans do. It needs a mathematical equation to build a scenario that represents the reality. The mathematical equation is a representation of the reality and usually simplifies the problem to be solved, due to that incorporates mistakes and has limitations to be generalized. Because of it, the application of machine learning and deep learning techniques to control vector-borne diseases must be designed and/or trained for this specific purpose. There is no such generic approach: each problem has its own specificity and therefore must be treated with exclusivity.

4.2 Robust dataset

Another important limitation of machine learning and deep learning is the need of historical data to be used for algorithm training, learn from these data, and predict a reliable outcome. The availability, disposal, and variability of these existing data are crucial for the computer learning process. "Objects in realistic settings exhibit considerable variability, so to learn to recognize them, it is necessary to use much larger training sets [6]."

Entomology, for instance, has small dataset size available open source, which turns to be difficult to adapt the model and solve the problem with proper accuracy and reliability. Researchers should be aware that the application of machine learning and deep learning for zoonotic diseases must consider the building of a robust dataset.

4.3 Underfitting and overfitting

Underfitting and overfitting also need to be addressed during the use of machine learning and deep learning techniques. The first one relies when small data are presented in the training or the training does not run a sufficient number of epochs (learning cycles). In this case, the mathematical model is unable to capture the features complexity of the input provided and present a high error level in the output—too many wrong predictions when new data are presented.

Overfitting relies when the data presented have small variability or the training learning cycles are too much, and instead of reducing the error after each epoch, it starts to increase. To clarify the understanding, imagine a student who, among the elementary arithmetic operations (addition, subtraction, division, and multiplication), only dominates multiplication. If a test is presented only with questions to multiply numbers, probably the student will have a good grade, but you cannot measure his/her knowledge with this test. That exactly what happens with the computer if the variability of data is low. The training result might present a high accuracy, but in the real world, it is not reliable.

Figure 10 graphically shows underfitting and overfitting—validation error represents the predicting error when new data are presented.

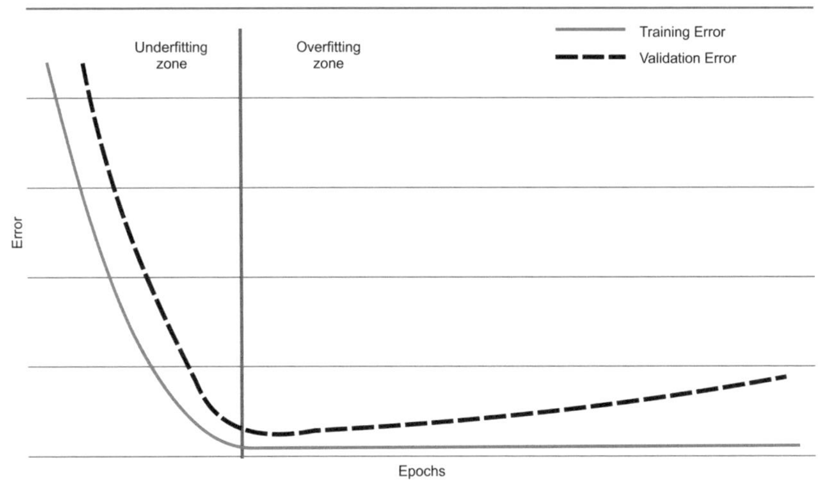

Figure 10.
Representation of underfitting and overfitting. "Adapted from [1]".

There are some methods to reduce overfitting. "The easiest and most common method is to artificially enlarge the dataset [6]."

5. Conclusions

Novel and important applications are available with the development of data mining methods. Artificial intelligence techniques are an important field to be applied on the control of vector-borne diseases. A complete and accurate identification of the 5000 mosquito's species that were already identified should be tested in this model as well as other species groups, such as complex or cryptic species, and in different populations of the same species.

Artificial intelligence could help to develop a system that anyone, who capture larvae or adult's mosquitos in several regions, can identify the *Aedes* mosquito. In the near future, a complete identification of any insect or new nonclassified ones that exist in this world could be automatically classified by anyone using a smartphone. AI will never replace mankind but will help to keep memories and activities that humans have discovered in our millenarian existence.

Acknowledgements

This project received financial support from Fundação de Amparo à Pesquisa do Estado da Bahia—FAPESB via scholarships. We are thankfull to Daniel André Dias Imperial Pereira and Alexandre Morais Cavalcanti, students at University Center SENAI/CIMATEC. We also thank Eduardo Oyama, entomologist from the Technology Institute of Health—SENAI CIMATEC, for supporting the work and sharing his experience. We are also in debt with the Department of Culicidae collection from Fiocruz Rio de Janeiro, especially Maycon Neves and Monique Motta from their staff.

Conflict of interest

We have no "conflict of interest."

Appendices and nomenclature

AI	artificial intelligence
ML	machine learning
DL	deep learning
ILSVRC	ImageNet large scale visual recognition challenge
WO	PCI patents (world)
CNN	convolutional neural networks
SVM	support vector machine

Author details

Daniel da Silva Motta[1]*, Roberto Badaró[2], Alex Santos[1] and Frank Kirchner[3]

1 University Center SENAI/CIMATEC, Salvador, Bahia, Brazil

2 Technology Institute of Health—SENAI CIMATEC, Salvador, Bahia, Brazil

3 Research Centre for Artificial Intelligence—DFKI, Bremen, Germany

*Address all correspondence to: dmotta@fieb.org.br

References

[1] Goodfellow I, Bengio Y, Courville A. Deep Learning [Internet]. Cambridge, Massachusetts, USA: MIT Press; 2016. Available from: http://www.deeplearningbook.org

[2] Yoav S, Perrault R, Brynjolfsson E, Jack C, Legassick C. Artificial Intelligence Index, 2017 Annual Report [Internet]. 2017. Available from: http://aiindex.org/2017-report.pdf

[3] Kajaree D, Behera R. A survey on machine learning: Concept, algorithms and applications. International Journal of Electronics Communication and Computer Engineering. 2017;**5**:1302-1309. DOI: 10.15680/IJIRCCE.2017

[4] De Souza VMA, Silva DF, Batista GEAPA. Classification of data streams applied to insect recognition: Initial results. In: Proc—2013 Brazilian Conf Intell Syst, BRACIS 2013. 2013. pp. 76-81. DOI: 10.1109/BRACIS.2013.21

[5] Silva DF, De Souza VMA, Batista GEAPA, Keogh E, Ellis DPW. Applying machine learning and audio analysis techniques to insect recognition in intelligent traps. In: Proceedings—2013 12th International Conference on Machine Learning and Applications, ICMLA 2013. 2013. pp. 99-104. DOI: 10.1109/ICMLA.2013.24

[6] Krizhevsky A, Sutskever I, Hinton GE. ImageNet classification with deep convolutional neural networks. Advances in Neural Information Processing Systems. 2012;**25**(2):1-9. DOI: 10.1016/j.protcy.2014.09.007

[7] WHO. Global Vector Control Response 2017-2030—Background Document to Inform Deliberations during the 70th Session of the World Health Assembly. WHO. 2017. p. 47

[8] Park SI, Bisgin H, Ding H, Semey HG, Langley DA, Tong W, et al. Species identification of food contaminating beetles by recognizing patterns in microscopic images of elytra fragments. PLoS One. 2016;**11**:1-22. DOI: 10.1371/journal.pone.0157940

[9] Pombi M, Guelbeogo WM, Calzetta M, Sagnon N, Petrarca V, La Gioia V, et al. Evaluation of a protocol for remote identification of mosquito vector species reveals BG-sentinel trap as an efficient tool for *Anopheles gambiae* outdoor collection in Burkina Faso. Malaria Journal. 2015;**14**:161. DOI: 10.1186/s12936-015-0674-7

[10] Ouyang TH, Yang EC, Jiang JA, Lin TT. Mosquito vector monitoring system based on optical wingbeat classification. Computers and Electronics in Agriculture. 2015;**118**:47-55. DOI: 10.1016/j.compag.2015.08.021

[11] Utsugi J, Toshihide K, Motomi ITO. Current progress in DNA barcoding and future implications for entomology. Entomological Science. 2011;**14**:107-124. DOI: 10.1111/j.1479-8298.2011.00449.x

[12] Karthika P, Vadivalagan C, Thirumurugan D, Kumar RR, Murugan K, Canale A, et al. DNA barcoding of five Japanese encephalitis mosquito vectors (*Culex fuscocephala*, *Culex gelidus*, *Culex tritaeniorhynchus*, *Culex pseudovishnui* and *Culex vishnui*). Acta Tropica. 2018;**183**:84-91. DOI: 10.1016/j.actatropica.2018.04.006

[13] Consoli RAGB, de Oliveira RL. Principais mosquitos de importância sanitária no Brasil. Rio de Janeiro, Brasil: Fundação Oswaldo Cruz; 1998. DOI: 10.1590/S0102-311X1995000100027

[14] Schaper S, Hernández-Chavarría F. Scanning electron microscopy of the four larval instars of the Dengue

fever vector *Aedes aegypti* (*Diptera*: *Culicidae*). Revista de Biología Tropical. 2006;**54**:847-852

[15] Kumar NP, Rajavel AR, Natarajan R, Jambulingam P. DNA barcodes can distinguish species of Indian mosquitoes (*Diptera*: *Culicidae*). Journal of Medical Entomology. 2007;**44**:1-7. DOI: 10.1603/0022-2585(2007)44[1:DBCDSO]2.0.CO;2

[16] Lorenz C, Sergio A, Suesdek L. Artificial neural network applied as a methodology of mosquito species identification. Acta Tropica. 2015;**152**:165-169. DOI: 10.1016/j.actatropica.2015.09.011

[17] Reyes AMMDL, Reyes ACA, Torres JL, Padilla DA, Villaverde J. Detection of Aedes Aegypti mosquito by digital image processing techniques and support vector machine. In: 2016 IEEE Region 10 Conference (TENCON). 2016. pp. 2342-2345. DOI: 10.1109/TENCON.2016.7848448

[18] Sanchez-Ortiz A, Fierro-Radilla A, Arista-Jalife A, Cedillo-Hernandez M, Nakano-Miyatake M, Robles-Camarillo D, et al. Mosquito larva classification method based on convolutional neural networks. In: 2017 International Conference on Electronics, Communications and Computers (CONIELECOMP). 2017. pp. 1-6. DOI: 10.1109/CONIELECOMP.2017.7891835